Keto Desserts Recipe Book

A Collection of Chaffles, Cookies and Cakes to Combine Diet and Good Taste

Kimberly Wood

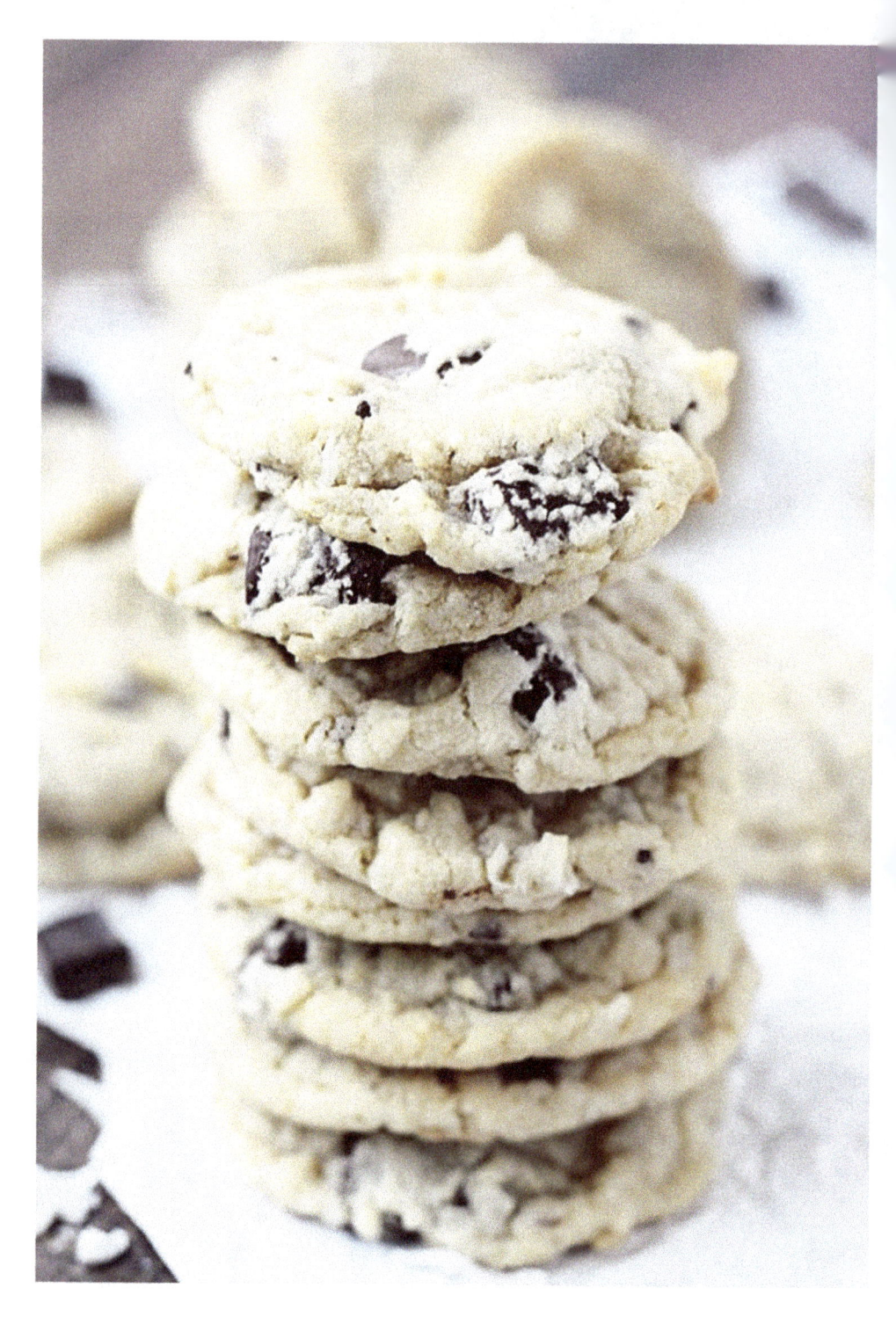

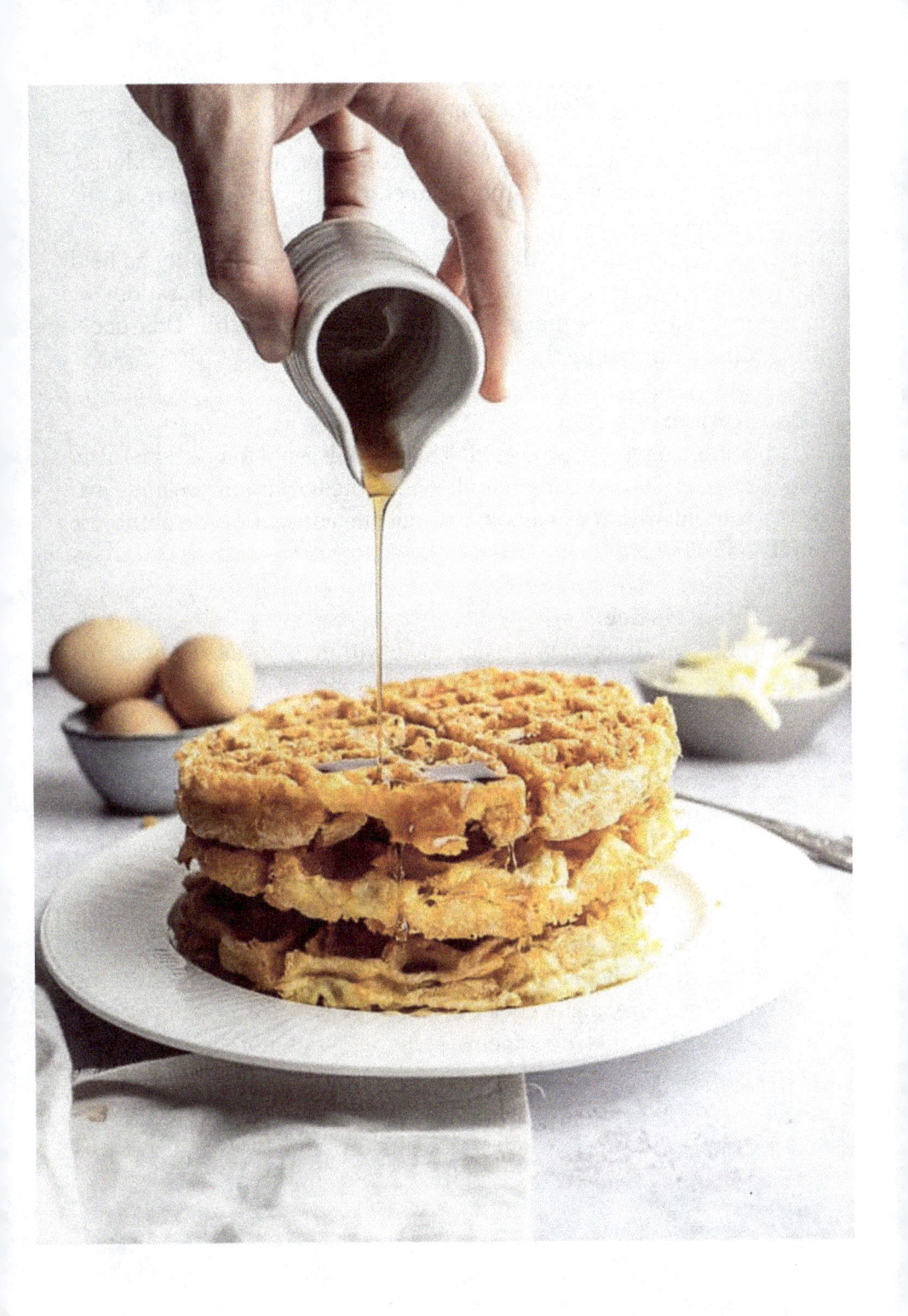

© Copyright 2021 – All rights reserved.

The content contained within this book may not be reproduced, duplicated or transmitted without direct written permission from the author or the publisher.
Under no circumstances will any blame or legal responsibility be held against the publisher, or author, for any damages, reparation, or monetary loss due to the information contained within this book. Either directly or indirectly.

Legal Notice:
This book is copyright protected. This book is only for personal use. You cannot amend, distribute, sell, use, quote or paraphrase any part, or the content within this book, without the consent of the author or publisher.

Disclaimer Notice:
Please note the information contained within this document is for educational and entertainment purposes only. All effort has been executed to present accurate, up to date, and reliable, complete information. No warranties of any kind are declared or implied. Readers acknowledge that the author is not engaging in the rendering of legal, financial, medical or professional advice. The content within this book has been derived from various sources. Please consult a licensed professional before attempting any techniques outlined in this book.
By reading this document, the reader agrees that under no circumstances is the author responsible for any losses, direct or indirect, which are incurred as a result of the use of information contained within this document, including, but not limited to, — errors, omissions, or inaccuracies.

Table of Contents

- BIRTHDAY CAKE CHAFFLE 7
- CHOCO CHAFFLE CAKE 9
- COCONUT CREAM CAKE CHAFFLE 13
- COFFEE CAKE 16
- CRUNCHY COCONUT CHAFFLES CAKE 18
- LEMON CHAFFLE CAKE 20
- NEW YEAR KETO CHAFFLE CAKE 22
- PEANUT BUTTER CHAFFLE CAKE 24
- STRAWBERRY SHORTCAKE CHAFFLE 28
- WHIPPED CREAM TOPPING 30
- CHAFFLES ICE CREAM TOPPING 31
- CHAFFLES WITH CHOCOLATE BALLS 32
- CHAFFLES WITH STRAWBERRY FROSTY 35
- CHERRY & CREAM TOPPED CHAFFLES 36
- CHOCOLATE CHAFFLE ROLLS 39
- CHOCOLATE CHIP CHAFFLES 41
- CHOCOLATE KETO CHAFFLE 43
- CINNAMON CHAFFLE ROLLS 45
- CREAMY CHAFFLES 47
- DELICIOUS YOGURT CHAFFLE 49
- DOUBLE CHOCOLATE CHAFFLES 51
- DOUBLE-DECKER CHAFFLE 53
- FRESH BLUEBERRY CHAFFLES 55
- ICE CREAM CHAFFLE 57
- KETO CHOCOLATE CHIP CANNOLI CHAFFLE 59
- OREO CHAFFLE 61
- PEANUT BUTTER CUP CHAFFLES 63
- PUMPKIN CHOCOLATE CHIP CHAFFLES 65

- Keto Marshmallow Creme Fluff Recipe 67
- Smores Chaffles 69
- Vanilla Twinkie Chaffle 71
- Walnut Low-Carb Chaffles 73
- Caramel Cake 74
- Carrot & Apple Spice Walnut Cake 78
- Chocolate-Lovers Cake 80
- Instant Pot Orange Rum Cake 82
- Keto Vanilla Pound Cake 84
- Pumpkin Caramel Bundt Cake 86
- Pumpkin Pie Spice Mug Cake 88
- Slow-Cooked Gingerbread Cake 90
- Tiramisu Layer Cake 92
- No-Bake Banana Split Cheesecake 95
- No-Bake Plain Cheesecake 97
- Almond Cinnamon Butter Cookies 99
- Amaretti Cookies 100
- Chocolate Chip Cookies 102
- Coconut Cookies 104
- Cranberry Bliss Cookies 106

Birthday Cake Chaffle

Servings Provided: 4

Nutritional Facts - Per Serving:

- Net Carbohydrates: 4.3 grams
- Calories: 141
- Protein: 4.7 grams
- Fats: 10.2 grams

Ingredients Needed:

- Eggs (2)
- Almond flour (.25 cup)
- Coconut flour (1 tsp.)
- Melted butter (2 tbsp.)
- Unchilled cream cheese (2 tbsp.)
- Cake batter extract (1 tsp.)
- Vanilla extract (.5 tsp.)
- Monk fruit/Swerve - confectioners sweetener (2 tbsp.)
- Xanthan powder (.25 tsp.)
- Baking powder (.5 tsp.)

Frosting Ingredients:

- Swerve confectioners sweetener/monk fruit (2 tbsp.)
- Heavy whipping cream (.5 cup)

- Vanilla extract (.5 tsp.)

Preparation Directions:
1. Warm a mini waffle maker.
2. Add all of the chaffle cake fixings into a blender, mixing using the high setting until it's smooth.
3. Wait a minute or two and add about two to three tablespoons of batter to the waffle maker and cook it for about two to three minutes until it's golden brown.
4. In another bowl, prepare the whipped cream vanilla frosting.
5. Add all of the components and combine it with a hand mixer until the whipping cream is thick and forms soft peaks.
6. Wait for the cake chaffles to cool completely before frosting the cake. If you frost it too soon, it will melt the frosting.

Choco Chaffle Cake

Servings Provided: 8

Nutritional Facts - Per Serving:

- Net Carbohydrates: 1.67 grams
- Calories: 243
- Protein: 7.87 grams
- Fats: 42.4 grams

Ingredients Needed:

- Keto chocolate chaffles (8)
- Keto-friendly peanut butter (2 cups)
- Raspberries (16 oz.)

Preparation Directions:

1. Prepare the chaffles. Use the chocolate chaffle recipe in chapter two.
2. Spread peanut butter over each chaffle and garnish with raspberries.
3. A great Christmas time idea!

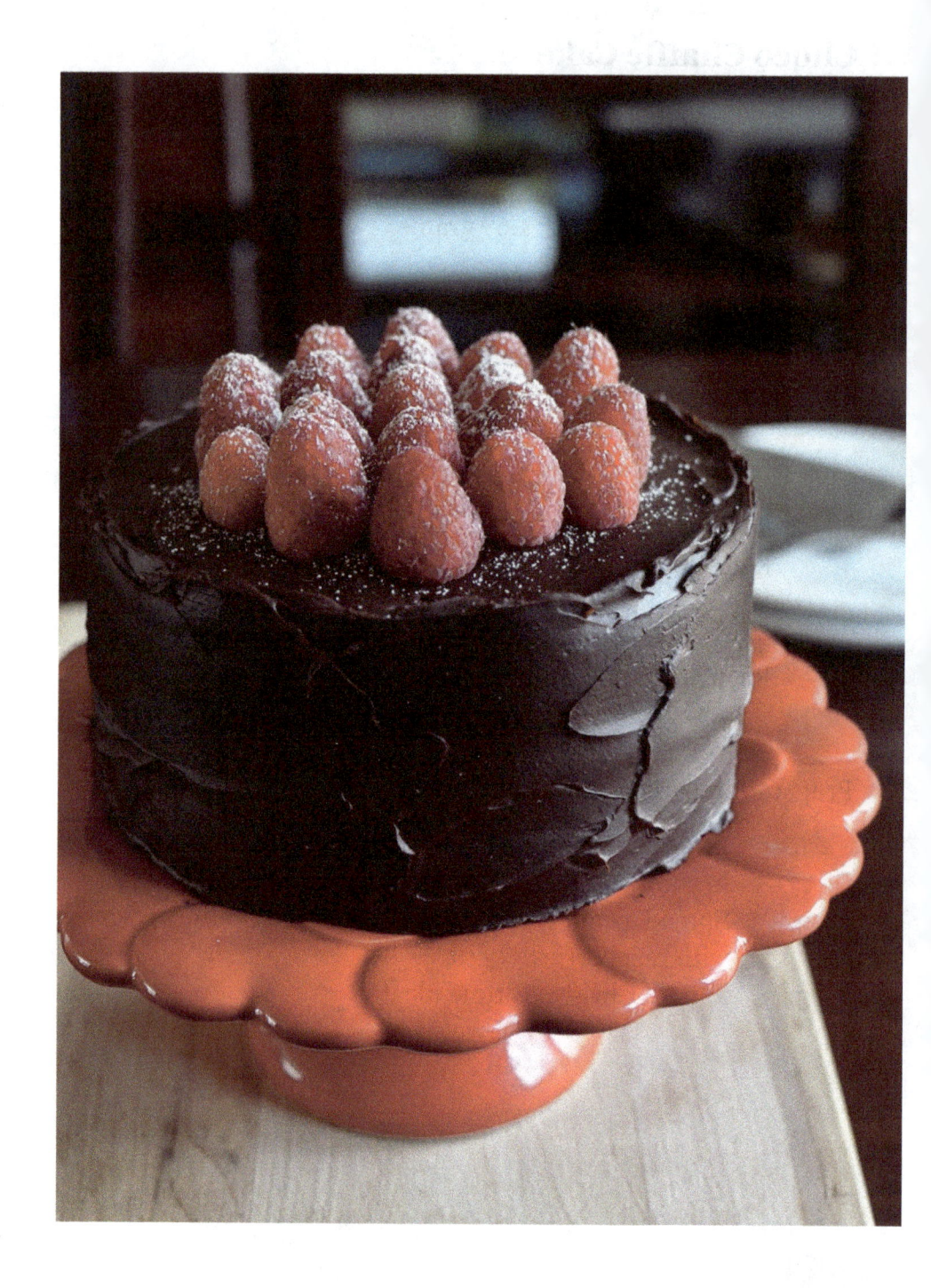

Chocolate Chaffle Cake With Cream Cheese Frosting

Servings Provided: 2 with the frosting

Nutritional Facts - Per Serving:
- Net Carbohydrates: 3 grams
- Calories: 151
- Protein: 6 grams
- Fats: 13 grams

Ingredients Needed:

Cake Ingredients:
- Cocoa powder (2 tbsp.)
- Swerve granulated sweetener (2 tbsp.)
- Egg (1)
- Baking powder (.25 tsp.)
- Heavy whipping cream (1 tbsp.)
- Vanilla extract (.5 tsp.)
- Almond flour (1 tbsp.)

Frosting Ingredients:
- Cream cheese (2 tbsp.)
- Swerve confectioners (2 tsp.)

- Vanilla extract (.125 tsp.)
- Heavy cream (1 tsp.)

Preparation Directions:

1. Whisk the almond flour, cocoa powder, swerve, and baking powder.
2. Mix in the vanilla extract and heavy whipping cream.
3. Whisk and add in the egg, scraping the sides of the bowl when it's needed.
4. Wait for three to four minutes while the mini waffle maker heats.
5. Add half of the batter to the wafflv maker and cook for approximately four minutes. Then cook the second waffle. While the second chocolate keto waffle is cooking, prepare the frosting.
6. In a small microwave-safe bowl, add two tablespoons of cream cheese. Microwave the cream cheese for eight seconds to soften it.
7. Add in heavy whipping cream and vanilla extract, using a small hand mixer.
8. Fold in the confectioners swerve.
9. Place one chocolate chaffle on a plate, top with a layer of frosting.
10. Put the second chocolate chaffle on top of the frosting layer, and spread the rest of the frosting on top.

Coconut Cream Cake Chaffle

Servings Provided: 4**

Nutritional Facts - Per Serving:

- Net Carbohydrates: 5 grams
- Calories: 157
- Protein: 5.1 grams
- Fats: 14.1 grams

Ingredients Needed:

Chaffles:

- Eggs (2)
- Unchilled cream cheese - softened (1 oz.)
- Finely shredded unsweetened coconut (2 tbsp.)
- Powdered sweetener blend - such as Swerve or Lakanto (2 tbsp.)
- Coconut oil/Melted butter (1 tbsp.)
- Coconut extract (.5 tsp.)
- Vanilla extract (.5 tsp.)

The Filling:

- Coconut milk (.33 cup)
- Unsweetened almond or cashew milk (.33 cup)
- Eggs yolks (2)

- Powdered sweetener blend- Swerve/Lakanto (2 tbsp.)
- Xanthan gum (.25 tsp.)
- Butter (2 tsp.)
- Salt (1 pinch)
- Finely shredded unsweetened coconut (.25 cup)

Optional:

- Sugar-free whipped cream
- Finely shredded unsweetened coconut - lightly toasted (1 tbsp.)

Preparation Directions:
1. Heat a mini waffle iron until thoroughly hot.
2. Beat each of the chaffle fixings in a small bowl.
3. Add a heaping two tablespoons of batter to the waffle iron and cook until nicely browned, and the waffle iron stops steaming (approx. five min.).
4. Note** Repeat three times to make four chaffles. You only need three for the recipe.
5. Prepare the filling. Heat the coconut and almond milk in a small saucepan using med-low heat (steaming hot, but not simmering or boiling).
6. In another bowl, lightly whisk the egg yolks. While whisking the milk constantly, slowly drizzle the egg yolks into the milk.
7. Heat, constantly stirring until the mixture thickens slightly. Don't boil.

8. Whisk in the sweetener. While constantly whisking, slowly sprinkle in the xanthan gum. Continue to cook for one minute.
9. Remove from the heat and add the remaining fixings.
10. Pour the filling into a container, cover the surface with plastic wrap and refrigerate until cool to prevent a skin from forming on the filling. The mixture will thicken as it cools.
1. 11. Spread ⅓ of the filling over three chaffles, stack them together to make a cake, top with whipped cream, and garnish with toasted coconut.

Coffee Cake

Servings Provided: 2 chaffles

Nutritional Facts - Per Serving - both chaffles:

- Net Carbohydrates: 3 grams
- Calories: 391
- Protein: 10 grams
- Fats: 35 grams

Ingredients Needed:

For the Chaffle:

- Butter (1 tbsp.)
- Egg (1)
- Vanilla (.5 tsp.)
- Almond flour (2 tbsp.)
- Coconut flour (1 tbsp.)
- Baking powder (.125 tsp.)
- Monk fruit (1 tbsp.)

For the Crumble:

- Cinnamon (.5 tsp.)
- Melted butter (1 tbsp.)
- Monk fruit/another sweetener (1 tsp.)
- Chopped pecans (1 tbsp.)

Preparation Directions:

1. Melt the butter in a bowl. Mix in the egg, vanilla, and the rest of the ingredients for the chaffle.
2. The Crumble: In another bowl with the melted butter for the crumble, add and mix the remainder of the fixings.
3. Pour half of the chaffle mix into your mini waffle maker/griddle.

2. Top it with half of the crumble mixture.
3. Cook five minutes or until done. Repeat with the other half of the ingredients.
4. Let the chaffle cool slightly before you spread the frosting.

Crunchy Coconut Chaffles Cake

Servings Provided: 4

Nutritional Facts - Per Serving:

- Net Carbohydrates: 0.26 grams
- Calories: 318
- Protein: 15.72 grams
- Fats: 26.05 grams

Ingredients Needed:

The Chaffles:

- Coconut flour (2 tbsp.)
- Stevia (1 tsp.)
- Coconut cream (2 tbsp.)
- Shredded cheese (1 cup)
- Large eggs (4)

The Toppings:

- Heavy cream (1 cup)
- Cherries (2 oz.)
- Blueberries (4 oz.)
- Raspberries (8 oz.)

Preparation Directions:

1. Prepare four mini chaffles using the chaffle fixings.
2. Heat the mini waffle maker until it is hot and add ¼ of the batter. Prepare the rest of the chaffles and let them cool slightly.

3. Spread heavy cream in each layer and top it off with the cherries, raspberries, and blueberries to serve.

Lemon Chaffle Cake

Servings Provided: 4 chaffles

Nutritional Facts - Per Serving:

- Net Carbohydrates: 3.9grams
- Calories: 221
- Protein: 5.6 grams
- Fats: 20.3 grams

Ingredients Needed:

Chaffle Cake:

- Unchilled cream cheese - softened (2 oz.)
- Eggs (2)
- Melted butter (2 tsp.)
- Coconut flour (2 tbsp.)
- Monk fruit powdered confectioners blend (1 tsp. + more if you like it sweeter)
- Baking powder (1 tsp.)
- Lemon extract (.5 tsp.)
- 20 drops cake batter extract 20 drops

Chaffle Frosting:

- Heavy whipping cream (.5 cup)
- Monk fruit powdered confectioners blend (1 tbsp.)

- Lemon extract (.25 tsp.)

Preparation Directions:
1. Preheat a mini waffle maker.
2. Add all of the ingredients for the chaffle cake in a blender and mix it until the batter is smooth (2 min.)
3. Use an ice cream scoop and fill the waffle iron with one full scoop
1. of batter (about three tablespoons).
4. While the chaffles are cooking, start making the frosting. In a medium-size bowl, add the chaffle frosting ingredients and mix until the frosting is thick with peaks.
5. Let the chaffles completely cool before frosting the cake.
6. Add lemon peel for extra flavor if desired.

New Year Keto Chaffle Cake

Servings Provided: 5

Nutritional Facts - Per Serving:

- Net Carbohydrates: 1.7 grams
- Calories: 243
- Protein: 7.9 grams
- Fats: 42.4 grams

Ingredients Needed:

- Almond flour (4 oz.)
- Cheddar cheese (2 cups)
- Eggs (5)
- Baking powder (2 tsp.)
- Stevia (1 tsp.)
- Melted almond butter (.25 cup)
- Vanilla extract (2 tsp.)
- Almond milk (3 tbsp.)
- Cranberries (1 cup)
- To Serve: Coconut cream (1 cup)

Preparation Directions:

1. Break the eggs in a bowl to whisk with the stevia, flour, and baking powder. Melt and fold in the butter until it's smooth.
2. Mix in the almond milk, cheese, vanilla, and cranberries.
3. Warm the waffle iron and lightly grease it using avocado oil.
4. Prepare the five chaffles in batches.
5. When ready, plate them and cover with the coconut cream. Slice and serve.

Peanut Butter Chaffle Cake

Servings Provided: 2

Nutritional Facts - Per Serving:

- Net Carbohydrates: 3 grams
- Calories: 92
- Protein: 5.5 grams
- Fats: 7 grams

Ingredients Needed:

- Sugar-Free Peanut Butter Powder (2 tbsp.)
- Monk fruit Confectioners Keto Sweetener (2 tbsp.)
- Egg (1)
- Baking Powder (.25 tsp.)
- Unchilled cream cheese - softened (1 tbsp.)
- Peanut Butter extract (.25 tsp.)

Frosting Ingredients

- Monk fruit Confectioners Keto Sweetener (2 tbsp.)
- Unchilled butter - softened (1 tbsp.)
- Sugar-free natural peanut butter/peanut butter powder (1 tbsp.)
- Unchilled cream cheese - softened (2 tbsp.)
- Vanilla (.25 tsp.)

Preparation Directions:

1. Whisk the egg and add the remaining ingredients, mixing until the batter is smooth.
2. Add the peanut butter extract (to add a more intense peanut butter flavor).
3. Pour half the batter into a preheated mini waffle maker and cook it for two to three minutes until it's crispy.
4. In another bowl, add the cream cheese, sweetener, sugar-free natural peanut butter, and vanilla. Mix the frosting until everything is well incorporated.
5. Spread or pipe the frosting on the waffle cake after it has completely cooled. Option 2: You can heat the frosting and add ½ teaspoon of water to make it a peanut butter glaze to drizzle over the peanut butter chaffle!

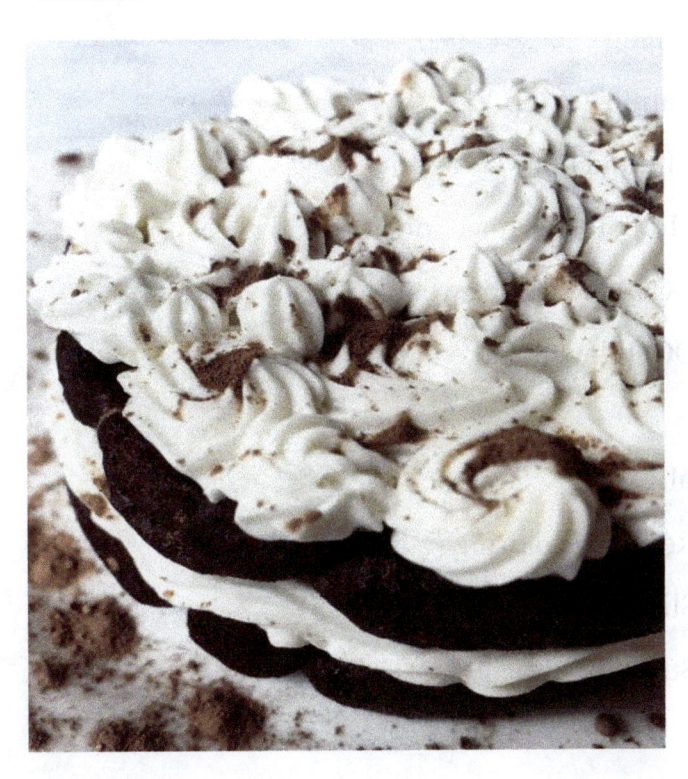

Strawberry Cake Chaffle

Servings Provided: 2

Nutritional Facts - Per Serving/Not counting the frosting:

- Net Carbohydrates: 2.6 grams
- Calories: 108
- Protein: 4.5 grams
- Fats: 7.9 grams

Ingredients Needed:

- Egg (1)
- Cream cheese (1 oz.)
- Vanilla (.5 tsp.)
- Almond flour (1 tbsp.)
- Monk fruit confectioners blend (1 tbsp.)
- OOOFlavors Strawberry Souffle (10 drops)
- OOOFlavors Cake Batter (10 drops)

Optional:

- Red food coloring (2 drops)
- Sliced strawberries (topping)
- Sugar-free sprinkles (as desired)

The Frosting:

- Unchilled cream cheese (1 tbsp.)
- Unchilled butter (1 tbsp.)
- Monk fruit confectioners blend (1 tbsp.)
- OOOFlavors Strawberry Souffle (9 drops)

Preparation Directions:

1. Whisk the egg until it's fluffy and mix with the rest of the chaffle fixings. Heat the mini waffle maker. Lightly grease and add half of the batter into the cooker. Cook it for about three minutes. Add the second half of the batter and cook it until browned.
2. Remove and cool both pieces. Prepare the frosting and frost the cooled chaffles. Top it off with berries and serve.

Strawberry Shortcake Chaffle

Servings Provided: 2 mini/1 regular

Nutritional Facts - Per Serving:

- Net Carbohydrates: 1 gram
- Calories: 112
- Protein: 7 grams
- Fats: 8 grams

Ingredients Needed:

The Topping:

- Fresh strawberries (3)
- Granulated swerve (.5 tbsp.)

Sweet Chaffle Ingredients:

- Almond flour (1 tbsp.)
- Mozzarella cheese (.5 cup)
- Egg (1)
- Granulated swerve (1 tbsp.)
- Vanilla extract (.25 tsp.)
- Keto Whipped Cream**

Preparation Directions:

1. Warm the mini waffle maker.

2. Rinse and chop the strawberries. Place them in a small bowl with
3. ½ tablespoon granulated swerve. Stir and set aside.
4. In another bowl, combine the almond flour, egg, mozzarella cheese, granulated swerve, and vanilla extract.
5. Dump ½ of the batter into the mini waffle maker and cook for three to four minutes. Then cook the other half of the batter for the second chaffle.
6. While your second chaffle is cooking, make your keto whipped cream if you do not have any on hand.
7. Assemble the two chaffles by placing whipped cream and strawberries on top with a drizzle of the juice.

Whipped Cream Topping

Servings Provided: 8

Nutritional Facts - Per Serving:

- Calories: 104
- Fats: 11 grams

Ingredients Needed:

- Heavy cream (1 cup)
- Pyure stevia (1 tbsp.)
- Vanilla extract (1 tsp.)

Preparation Directions:
1. Combine the stevia and cream in a mixer.
2. Whisk until it forms stiff peaks.
3. Lower the speed and add in the vanilla until it's just combined.

Chaffles Ice Cream Topping

Servings Provided: 2

Nutritional Facts - Per Serving:

- Net Carbohydrates: grams
- Calories: 263
- Protein: 16.26 grams
- Fats: 20.98 grams

Ingredients Needed:

- Coconut flour (1 cup)
- Frozen coconut cream (.25 cup)
- Strawberry chunks (.25 cup)
- Chocolate flakes (1 oz.)
- Vanilla extract (1 tsp.)
- Chaffles (4)

Preparation Directions:
1. Whisk each of the fixings in a bowl.
2. Spread the mixture between two chaffles and freeze for two hours before serving.

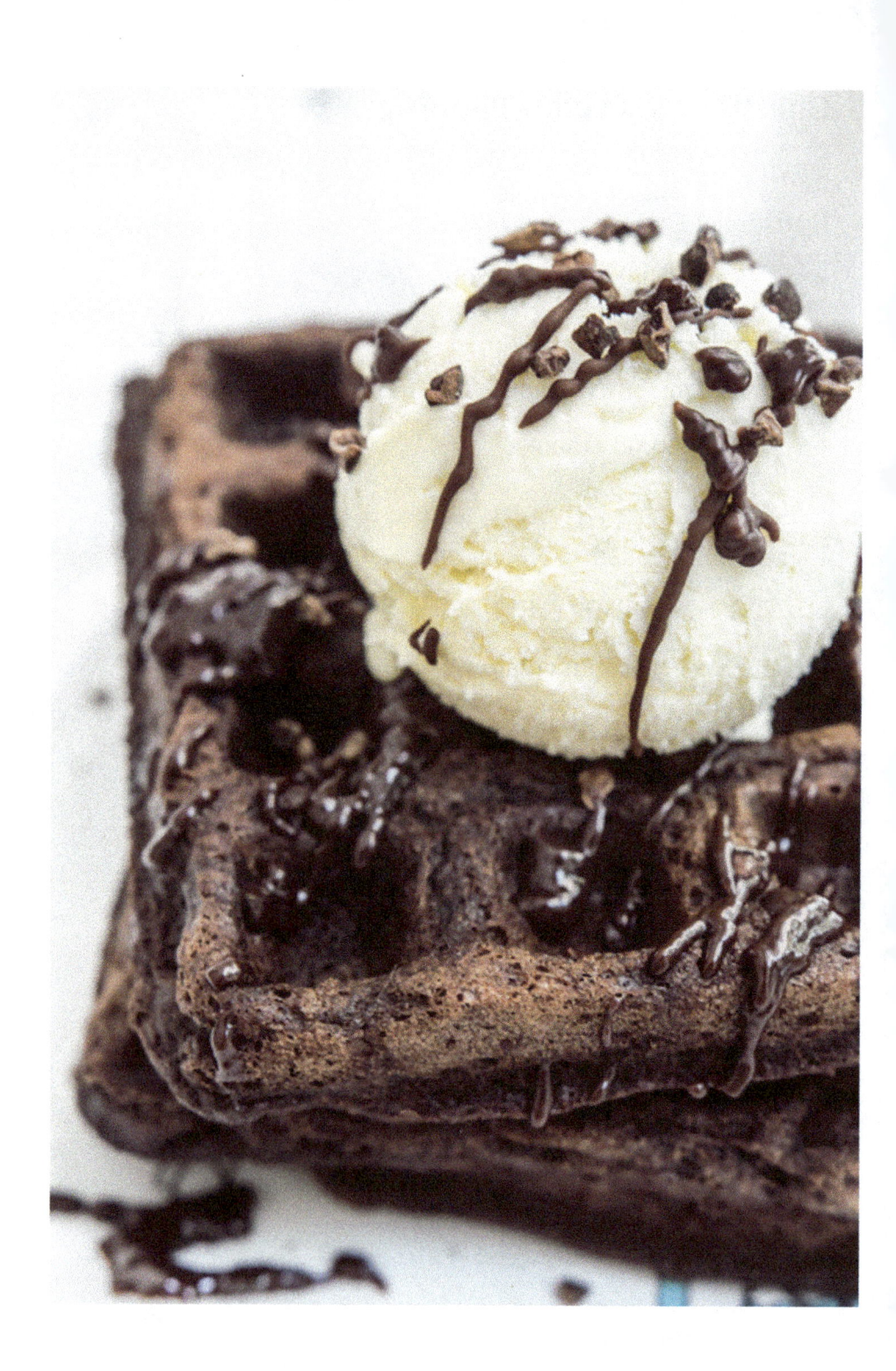

Chaffles With Chocolate Balls

Servings Provided: 2

Nutritional Facts - Per Serving:

- Net Carbohydrates: 0.42 grams
- Calories: 253
- Protein: 11.34 grams
- Fats: 22.15 grams

Ingredients Needed:

The Chaffle Ingredients:

- Mozzarella cheese (.5 cup)
- Egg (1)

The Ball of Chocolate:

- Heavy cream (.25 cup)
- Unsweetened cocoa powder (.5 cup)
- Coconut meat (.25 cup)

Preparation Directions:

1. Preheat the mini waffle iron and lightly mist it using a nonstick baking spray.
2. Prepare the chaffles in batches until browned and crispy (2-3 min.).

3. Make the chocolate balls and pop them into the freezer for about two hours.
4. Once they are set, serve with the chaffles for a delicious treat at any time.

Chaffles With Strawberry Frosty

Servings Provided: 2

Nutritional Facts - Per Serving:

- Net Carbohydrates: 0.95 grams
- Calories: 142
- Protein: 1.09 grams
- Fats: 11.22 grams

Ingredients Needed:

- Frozen strawberries (1 cup)
- Protein powder (1 scoop)
- Heavy cream (.5 cup)
- Stevia (1 tsp.)
- Chaffles (3)

Preparation Directions:

1. Whisk the fixings in a mixing container. Freeze the mixture for four hours or until it is set.
2. Top off the chaffles and serve.

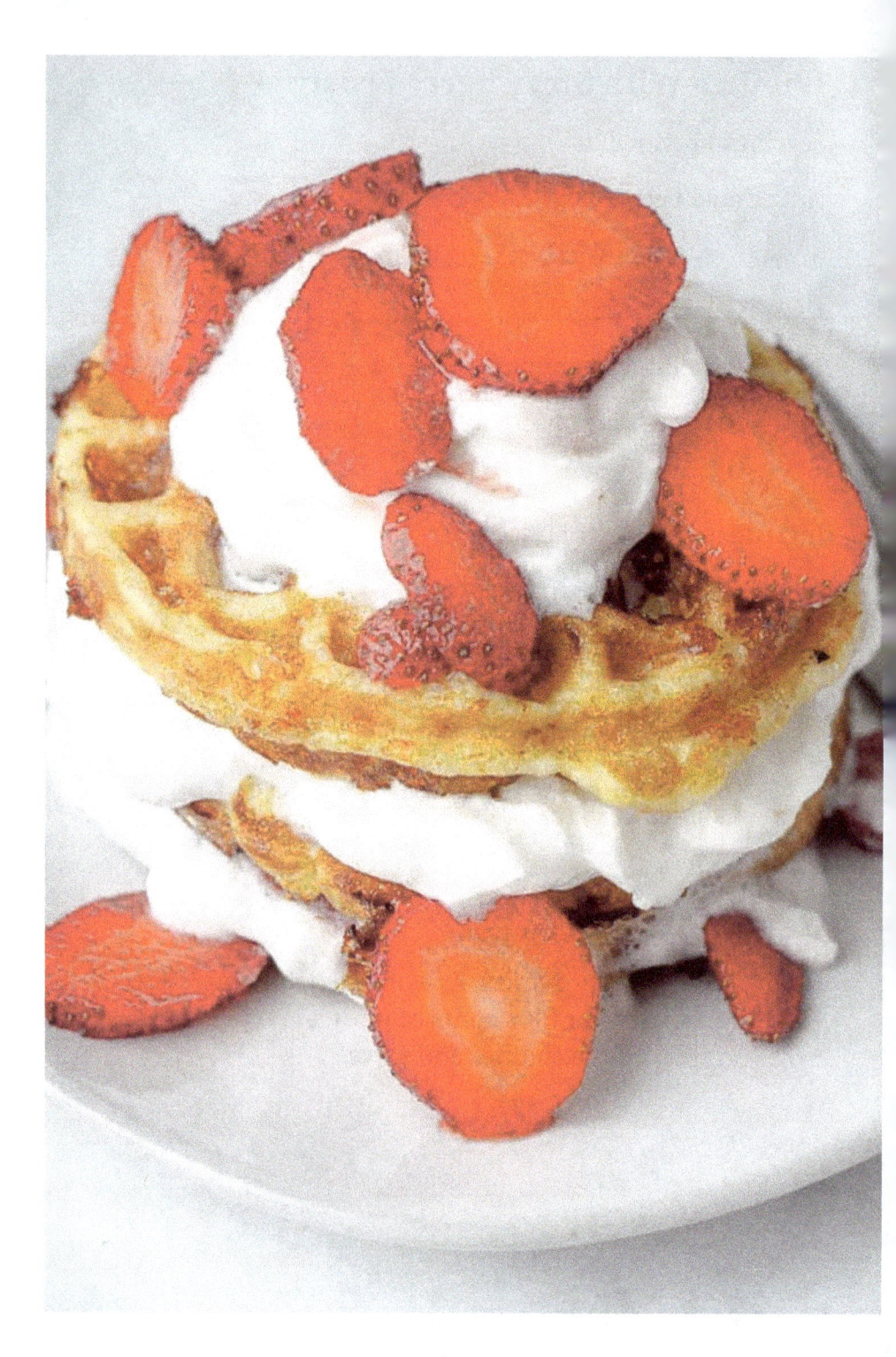

Cherry & Cream Topped Chaffles

Servings Provided: 4

Nutritional Facts - Per Serving:

- Net Carbohydrates: 2.34 grams
- Calories: 357
- Protein: 32.01 grams
- Fats: 22.6 grams

Ingredients Needed:

- Egg whites (1 cup)
- Baking powder (1 tsp.)
- Grated mozzarella cheese (1 cup)
- Vanilla (.5 tsp.)

The Toppings:

- Cherries (as desired - count carbs)
- Frozen heavy cream (.5 cup)

Preparation Directions:

1. Start a square waffle maker to preheat and spritz it using a non- stick cooking spray.
2. Use an electric mixer to beat the eggs until they are fluffy. Mix in the vanilla, baking powder, and cheese.

3. Pour the batter into the waffle maker in batches. Cook each batch for about three minutes.
4. Serve with the heavy cream and cherries for the toppings.

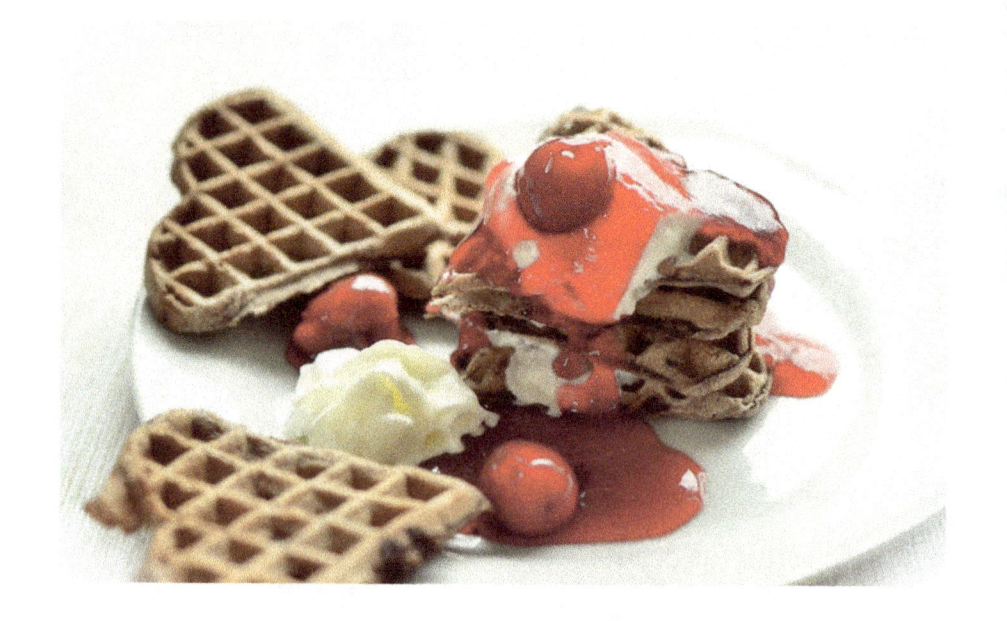

Chocolate Chaffle Rolls

Servings Provided: 2

Nutritional Facts - Per Serving:

- Net Carbohydrates: 1.38 grams
- Calories: 156
- Protein: 12.32 grams
- Fats: 10.62 grams

Ingredients Needed:

The Chaffles:

- Mozzarella cheese (.5 cup)
- Almond flour (1 tbsp.)
- Cinnamon (1 tsp.)
- Egg (1)
- Stevia (1 tsp.)

The Filling:

- Coconut cream (1 tbsp.)
- Keto-friendly chocolate chips (.25 cup)
- Coconut flour (1 tbsp.)

Preparation Directions:

1. Preheat a mini waffle iron. Lightly spray it using a cooking oil spray.
2. Whisk the chaffle ingredients and dump them into the waffle maker in batches. Cook them for three to four minutes.
3. Meanwhile, combine the cream, chocolate chips, and flour. Microwave it for 30 seconds. Spread the filling over the chaffles, roll it, and serve.

Chocolate Chip Chaffles

Servings Provided: 1

Nutritional Facts - Per Serving:

- Net Carbohydrates: 3 grams
- Calories: 304
- Protein: 17 grams
- Fats: 16 grams

Ingredients Needed:

- Egg (1 large)
- Coconut flour (1 tsp.)
- Monk fruit sweetener - ex Lakanto (1 tsp.)
- Vanilla extract (.5 tsp.)
- Finely shredded mozzarella (.5 cup)
- Sugar-free chocolate chips (2 tbsp.)

Preparation Directions:

1. Start the waffle iron to preheat.
2. Whisk the egg, coconut flour, sweetener, and vanilla.
3. Stir in the shredded cheese.
4. Spoon half of the batter into the waffle iron and dot with half of the chocolate chips. Spread a bit of batter over each chocolate chip.

5. Close the waffle iron and cook for three to four minutes or until as crispy as you'd like. Repeat with the remaining batter.
6. Serve hot with whipped cream or low-carb ice cream.

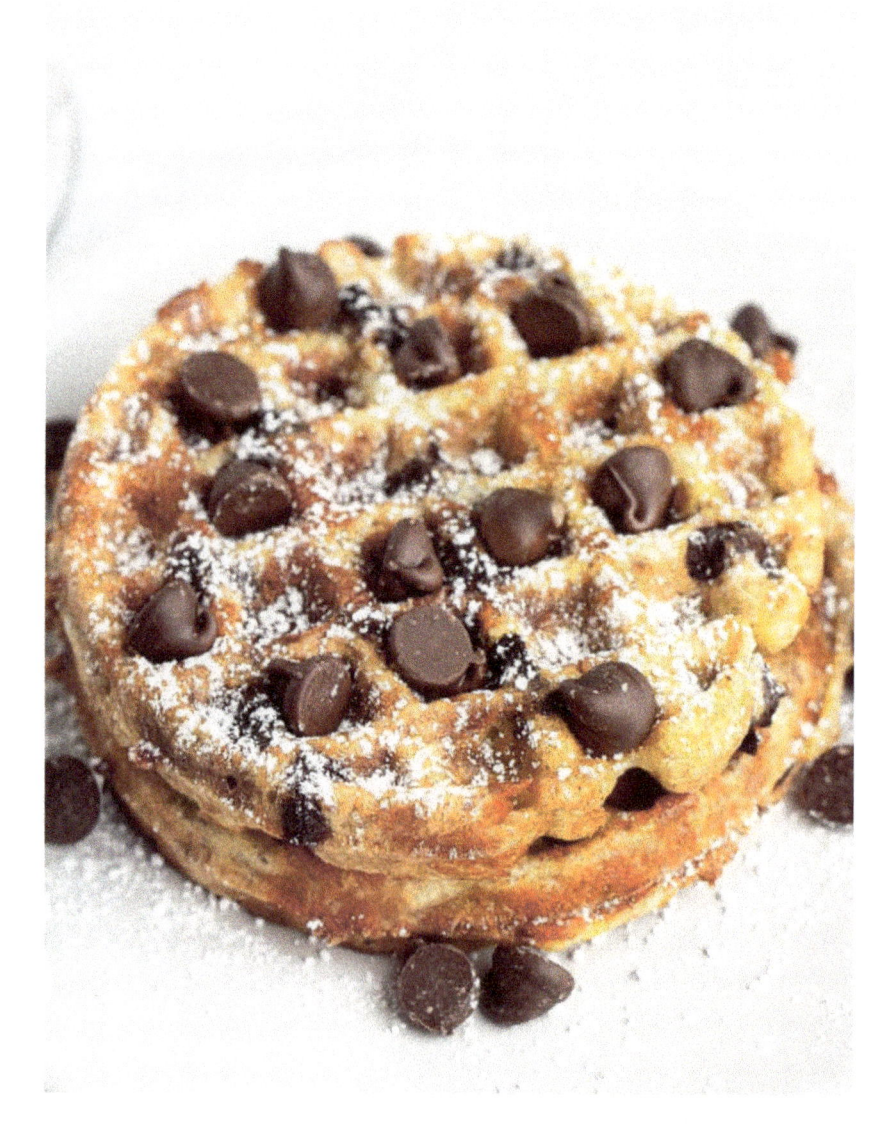

Chocolate Keto Chaffle

Servings Provided: 1 cake

Nutritional Facts - Per Serving:

- Net Carbohydrates: 7 grams
- Calories: 466
- Protein: 15 grams
- Fats: 44 grams

Ingredients Needed:

Dry Ingredients

- Almond flour (.25 cup)
- Cocoa powder (unsweetened (1 tbsp.)
- Erythritol (1.5 tbsp.)
- Baking powder (.5 tsp.)

Wet Ingredients:

- Egg (1 large)
- Butter/coconut oil - melted (2 tbsp.)
- Optional: Vanilla extract (.5 tsp.)
- Almond milk - unsweetened (.25 cup)

Preparation Directions:

1. Warm the waffle iron and melt the butter in the microwave.
2. Whisk the dry fixings in a bowl to remove the lumps.
3. Mix in the melted butter, almond milk, and whisked egg.
4. Pour the batter into the mini iron and cook for about 10 minutes.
5. Open the waffle iron and serve.

Cinnamon Chaffle Rolls

Servings Provided: 2

Nutritional Facts - Per Serving:

- Net Carbohydrates: 1.42 grams
- Calories: 210
- Protein: 12.72 grams
- Fats: 15.99 grams

Ingredients Needed:

The Chaffle:

- Almond flour (1 tbsp.)
- Mozzarella cheese (.5 cup)
- Egg (1)
- Cinnamon (1 tsp.)
- Stevia (1 tsp.)

The Glaze:

- Butter (1 tbsp.)
- Cream cheese (1 tbsp.)
- Cinnamon (1 tsp.)
- Vanilla extract (.25 tsp.)
- Coconut flour (1 tbsp.)

Preparation Directions:

1. Set the mini waffle iron to preheat. Lightly spritz it with cooking oil spray.
2. Whisk the chaffle ingredients.
3. Prepare the batter in batches, cooking them for three to four minutes.
4. Whisk the glaze ingredients. Spread it over the chaffle and roll the chaffle to serve.

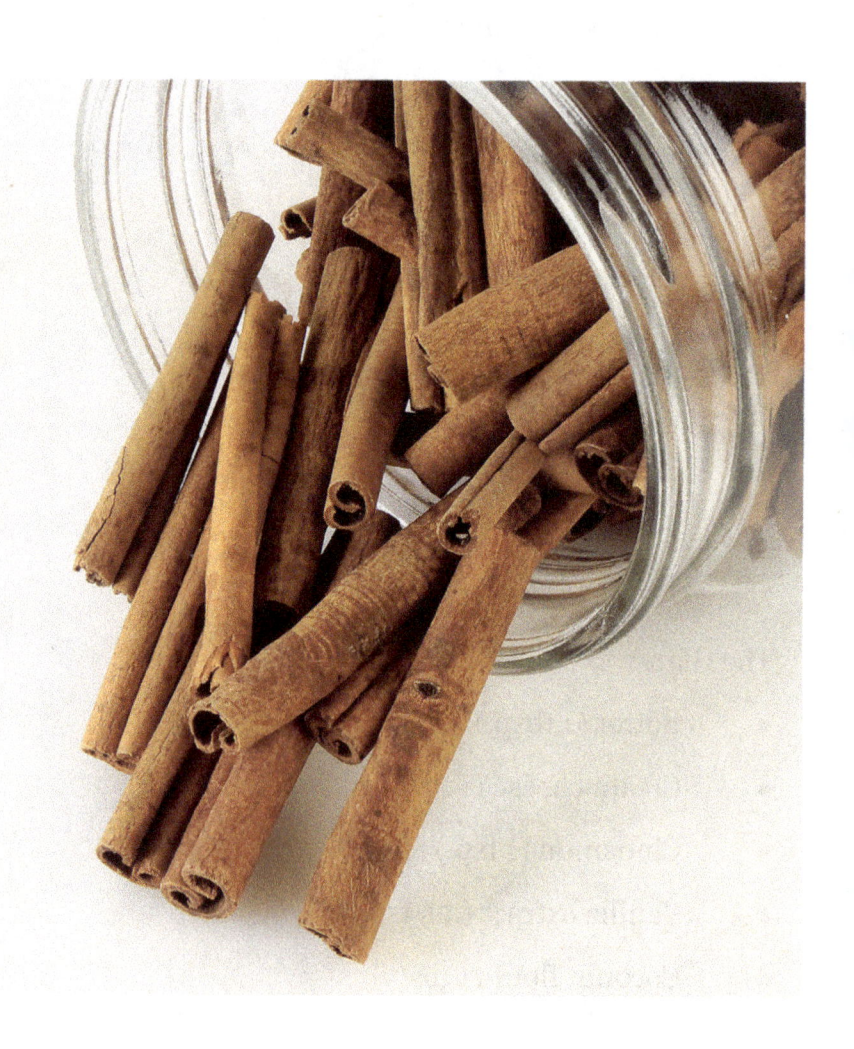

Creamy Chaffles

Servings Provided: 4

Nutritional Facts - Per Serving:

- Net Carbohydrates: 0.59 grams
- Calories: 263
- Protein: 16.26 grams
- Fats: 20.98 grams

Ingredients Needed:

The Chaffles:

- Egg whites (1 cup)
- Shredded cheddar cheese (1 cup)
- Cocoa powder (2 oz.)
- Salt (1 pinch)

The Garnish:

- Cream cheese (4 oz.)
- Blueberries
- Strawberries
- Coconut flour

Preparation Directions:

1. Whisk the eggs using an el ectric mixer until they are fluffy.
2. Toss in the cheese, salt, and cocoa powder.
3. Warm the waffle iron and spray with a cooking oil spray.
4. Pour in the batter in batches and cook for five minutes.
5. Serve with the cream cheese blueberries, strawberries, and coconut flour.

Delicious Yogurt Chaffle

Servings Provided: 4

Nutritional Facts - Per Serving:

- Net Carbohydrates: 1.59 grams
- Calories: 133
- Protein: 10.02 grams
- Fats: 9.75 grams

Ingredients Needed:

- Shredded mozzarella cheese (.5 cup)
- Shredded cheddar cheese (.5 cup)
- Egg (1)
- Ground almonds (2 tbsp.)
- Baking powder (.25 tsp.)
- Psyllium husk (1 tsp.)
- Greek yogurt (1 tbsp.)

The Topping:

- Frozen heavy cream (1 ice cream scoop)
- Frozen raspberry puree (1 scoop)
- Raspberries (2)

Preparation Directions:

1. Preheat the mini waffle iron and combine the fixings for the chaffles. Let the batter rest, and wait for about five minutes.
2. Lightly mist the grids using a cooking oil spray.
3. Sprinkle a portion of cheese onto the chaffle maker and pour in the first portion of batter.
4. Close the lid and cook for about four to five minutes.
5. Serve with a frozen scoop of the toppings.

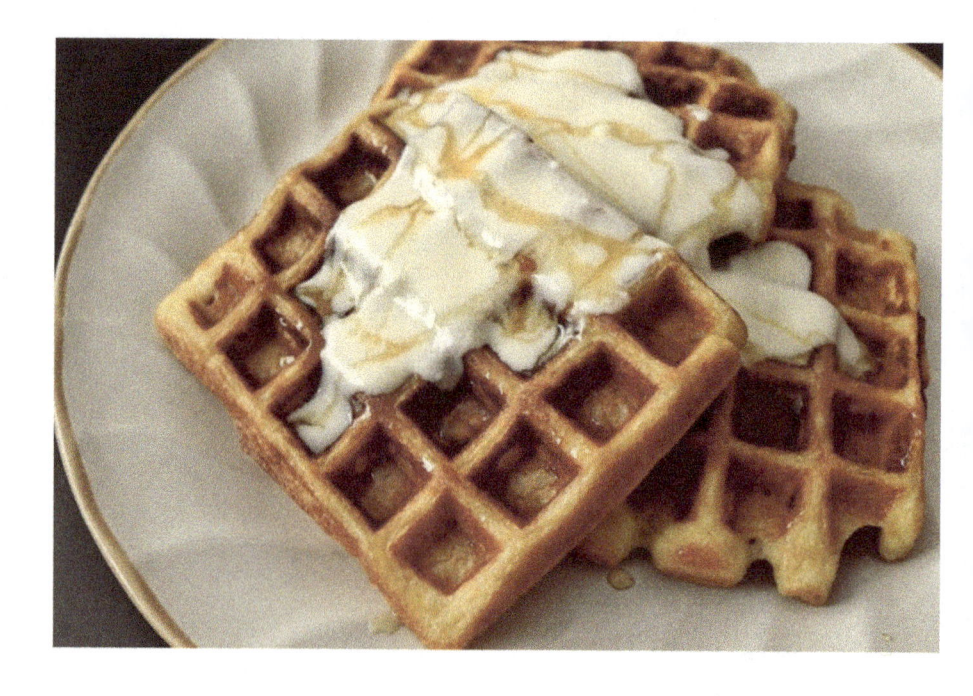

Double Chocolate Chaffles

Servings Provided: 2

Nutritional Facts - Per Serving:

- Net Carbohydrates: 2.59 grams
- Calories: 188
- Protein: 22.84 grams
- Fats: 8.28 grams

Ingredients Needed:

- Unsweetened chocolate chips (.25 cup)
- Cocoa powder (2 tbsp.)
- Egg whites (1 cup)
- Coffee powder (1 tsp.)
- Almond flour (2 tbsp.)
- Mozzarella cheese (.5 cup)
- Coconut milk (1 tbsp.)
- Baking powder (1 tsp.)
- Stevia (1 tsp.)

Preparation Directions:
1. Preheat the Belgian waffle maker.
2. Lightly spray the grids using a cooking spray.

3. Use an el ectric mixer to beat the eggs until they are creamy-white and fluffy.
4. Toss in the rest of the fixings. Mix it thoroughly.
5. Prepare the chaffles for about four to five minutes until golden brown.
6. Serve with a portion of coconut cream and berries.

Double-Decker Chaffle

Servings Provided: 2

Nutritional Facts - Per Serving:

- Net Carbohydrates: 2.37 grams
- Calories: 333
- Protein: 19.33 grams
- Fats: 24.83 grams

Ingredients Needed:

- Shredded cheese (1 cup)
- Egg (1 large)

The Topping:

- Chocolate balls (above recipe)
- Cranberry puree (4 oz.)
- Blueberries (2 oz.)
- Cranberries (2 oz.)

Preparation Directions:

1. Heat the mini waffle maker until it's hot.
2. Mix the chaffle batter and prepare the two chaffles. Cook them in two batches for 3-4 minutes.
3. Prepare the chocolate ball using the recipe in this chapter (Chaffles With Chocolate Balls).

4. Pop the chocolate ball, cranberries, and blueberries in the freezer for about two hours.
5. Serve by placing the chocolate ball between the two chaffles and topping it off with the berries.

Double-Decker Chaffle

Servings Provided: 2

Nutritional Facts - Per Serving:

- Net Carbohydrates: 2.37 grams
- Calories: 333
- Protein: 19.33 grams
- Fats: 24.83 grams

Ingredients Needed:

- Shredded cheese (1 cup)
- Egg (1 large)

The Topping:

- Chocolate balls (above recipe)
- Cranberry puree (4 oz.)
- Blueberries (2 oz.)
- Cranberries (2 oz.)

Preparation Directions:

1. Heat the mini waffle maker until it's hot.
2. Mix the chaffle batter and prepare the two chaffles. Cook them in two batches for 3-4 minutes.
3. Prepare the chocolate ball using the recipe in this chapter (Chaffles With Chocolate Balls).

4. Pop the chocolate ball, cranberries, and blueberries in the freezer for about two hours.
5. Serve by placing the chocolate ball between the two chaffles and topping it off with the berries.

Fresh Blueberry Chaffles

Servings Provided: 5

Nutritional Facts - Per Serving:

- Net Carbohydrates: 2 grams
- Calories: 116
- Protein: 8 grams
- Fats: 8 grams

Ingredients Needed:

- Mozzarella cheese (1 cup)
- Almond flour (2 tbsp.)
- Baking powder (1 tsp.)
- Eggs (2)
- Swerve (2 tsp.)
- Cinnamon (1 tsp.)
- Blueberries (3 tbsp.)
- Topping: Keto-friendly syrup/Swerve confectioners' sugar

Preparation Directions:

1. Heat the mini waffle cooker. Lightly spritz the waffle iron using a bit of cooking oil spray.
2. Combine all of the fixings.
3. Work in batches to prepare the chaffles.

4. Close the lid to cook for three to five minutes, checking them at the 3-minute mark for crispiness. If it is not ready, close the lid for another one to two minutes.
5. Garnish as desired.

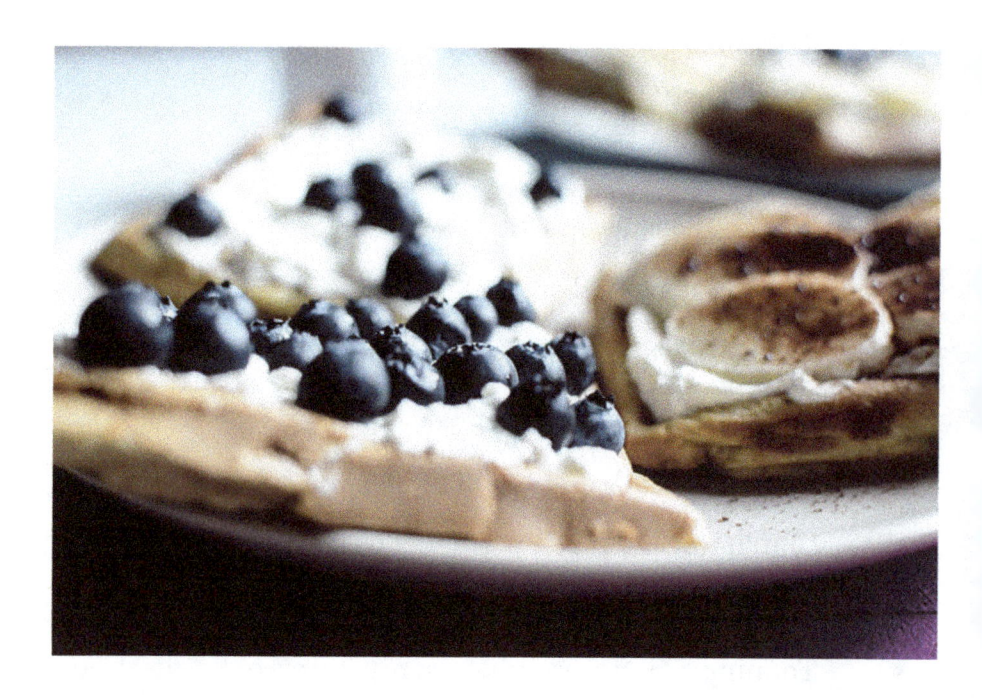

Ice Cream Chaffle

Servings Provided: 2

Nutritional Facts - Per Serving:

- Net Carbohydrates: 1 gram
- Calories: 273
- Protein: 11.42 grams
- Fats: 24.61 grams

Ingredients Needed:

The Batter:

- Egg (1)
- Baking powder (.5 tsp.)
- Almond flour (1 tbsp.)
- Shredded cheddar cheese (.5 cup)

To Serve:

- Keto-friendly chocolate chips
- Heavy cream (.5 cup)
- Blueberries (2 oz.)
- Raspberries (2 oz.)

Preparation Directions:

1. Set the mini waffle iron on to preheat.
2. Whisk the chaffle fixings to make two chaffles.
3. Prepare the ice cream ball by mixing the cream and chocolate chips. Place them in silicone molds and freeze for about two to four hours.
4. To Serve: Set the ice cream balls onto the chaffles and top with the berries.

Keto Chocolate Chip Cannoli Chaffle

Servings Provided: 4

Nutritional Facts - Per Serving:

- Net Carbohydrates: 1.8 grams

Ingredients Needed:

- Melted butter (1 tbsp.)
- Golden Monk fruit sweetener (1 tbsp.)
- Egg yolk (1)
- Vanilla Extract (.125 tsp.)
- Almond flour (3 tbsp.)
- Baking powder (.125 tsp.)
- Chocolate chips - sugar-free (1 tbsp.)

Topping Ingredients:

- Cream cheese (2 oz.)
- Confectioners sweetener - low-carb (2 tbsp.)
- Ricotta - full fat (6 tbsp.)
- Vanilla extract (.25 tsp.)
- Lemon extract (5 drops)

Preparation Directions:

1. Preheat the mini waffle maker.

2. In a small bowl, combine all of th e chaffle ingredients.
3. Place half of the ingredients in the mini waffle maker. Cook the chaffle for about three to four minutes.
4. While the chaffle is cooking, prepare the cannoli topping.
5. Add all of the cannoli toppings in a blender and mix until it's smooth and creamy.
6. Make your delicious treat when the chaffle is crispy.

Oreo Chaffle

Servings Provided: 3

Nutritional Facts - Per Serving:

- Net Carbohydrates: 2 grams
- Calories: 69
- Protein: 3.5 grams
- Fats: 5 grams

Ingredients Needed:

- Egg (1)
- Unsweetened Cocoa (1.5 tbsp.)
- Lakanto Monk fruit/choice of sweetener (2 tbsp.)
- Heavy cream (1 tbsp.)
- Coconut flour (1 tsp.)
- Baking powder (.5 tsp.)
- Vanilla (.5 tsp.)
- The Filling: Whipped cream

Preparation Directions:

1. Preheat a mini waffle maker.
2. In a small bowl, combin e each of the chaffle ingredients.
3. Pour half of the chaffle mixture into the center of the waffle iron. Cook it for three to five minutes.

4. Carefully remove and repeat the process for the second chaffle. Wait for a few minutes for them to crisp.
5. Serve with whipped cream in the center of the two chaffles for a real treat.

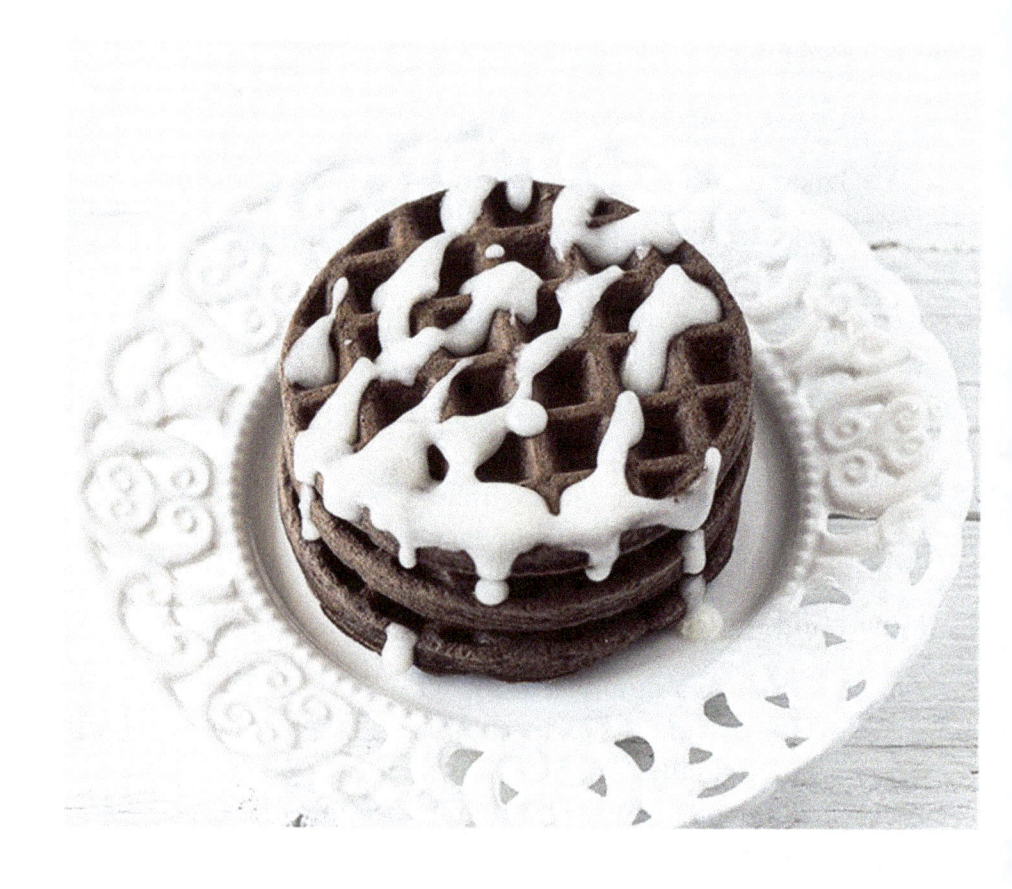

Peanut Butter Cup Chaffles

Servings Provided: 1

Nutritional Facts - Per Serving:

- Net Carbohydrates: 3 grams
- Calories: 210
- Protein: 8 grams
- Fats: 15 grams

Ingredients Needed:

The Chaffle:

- Egg (1 large)
- Cocoa powder (2 tbsp.)
- Sweetener of choice (1 tbsp.)
- Sugar-free chocolate chips (1 tbsp.)
- Espresso powder (.25 tsp.)
- Finely shredded mozzarella (.5 cup)

The Filling:

- Creamy peanut butter (3 tbsp.)
- Powdered sweetener (2 tbsp.)
- Unchilled butter - softened (1 tbsp.)

Preparation Directions:

1. Preheat the waffle iron.
2. Whisk the egg, cocoa powder, sweetener, chocolate chops, and espresso powder. Stir in the mozzarella.
3. Add half of the batter to the waffle maker and cook for about three minutes. Repeat with the remaining batter.
4. Meanwhile, add all of the filling ingredients to a small

1. Bowl and stir with a fork until it's smooth and creamy.
5. Let waffles cool before spreading with the peanut butter and closing to form a sandwich.

Pumpkin Chocolate Chip Chaffles

Servings Provided: 3

Nutritional Facts - Per Serving:

- Net Carbohydrates: 1 gram
- Calories: 93
- Protein: 7 grams
- Fats: 7 grams

Ingredients Needed:

- Shredded mozzarella cheese (.5 cup)
- Pumpkin puree (4 tsp.)
- Egg (1)
- Granulated swerve (2 tbsp.)
- Pumpkin pie spice (.25 tsp.)
- Sugar-free chocolate chips (4 tsp.)
- Almond flour (1 tbsp.)

Preparation Directions:
1. Preheat the mini waffle maker.
2. In a small bowl, whisk the pumpkin puree and egg. Add in the mozzarella cheese, almond flour, swerve and pumpkin spice and mix well.
3. Fold in the sugar-free chocolate chips
4. Add half of the chaffle mix to the waffle maker at a time. Cook it for four minutes.

5. DO NOT open before the four minutes is up. After that, you can open it to check it and make sure it is cooked all the way.
6. When the first one is completely done cooking, cook the second one.
7. Enjoy with some swerve confectioners sweetener or whipped cream on top.

Keto Marshmallow Creme Fluff Recipe

Servings Provided: 1 cup/16 tbsp.

Nutritional Facts - Per Serving:

- Net Carbohydrates: 0.4 grams
- Calories: 14
- Protein: 0.1 grams
- Fats: 1.4 grams

Ingredients Needed:

- Swerve confectioners (.5 cup)
- Pure vanilla extract (1 tsp.)
- Pink salt (1 pinch)
- Xanthan gum (1 tsp.)
- Heavy whipping cream (.5 cup)

Preparation Directions:

1. Prepare the fixings in a mixing bowl, except for the whipping cream.
2. Add half a cup of Swerve/another powdered sweetener you like.
3. Pour the heavy whipping cream over the sweetener.
4. Add the vanilla and pinch of salt. Whip it with a mixer until fluffy like whipped cream.
5. Sprinkle a small amount of the xanthan gum over it at a time, folding and mixing with a spatula.

6. Keep sprinkling and folding until the mixture becomes sticky and thick.
7. Store in the refrigerator.

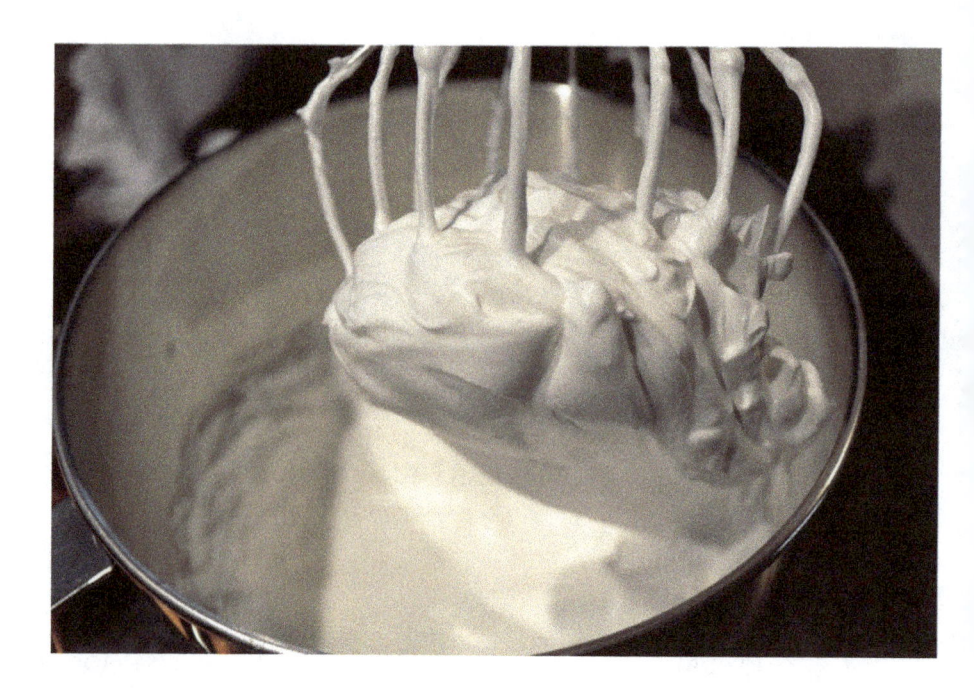

Smores Chaffles

Servings Provided: 2 pieces

Nutritional Facts - Per Serving:
- Net Carbohydrates: 2.9 grams
- Calories: 120
- Protein: 8.3 grams
- Fats: 8.1 grams

Ingredients Needed:
- Egg (1 large)
- Mozzarella cheese, shredded (.5 cup)
- Vanilla extract (.5 tsp.)
- Brown swerve (2 tbsp.)
- Optional: Psyllium Husk Powder (.5 tbsp.)
- Baking powder (.25 tsp.)
- Pink salt (1 pinch)
- Lily's Original Dark Chocolate Bar (¼ of 1)
- Keto Marshmallow Creme Fluff Recipe - see below (2 tbsp.)

Preparation Directions:
1. Make the batch of Keto Marshmallow Creme Fluff.

2. Whisk the egg until creamy. Add vanilla and brown swerve, mixing well.
3. Stir in the shredded cheese and fold in the psyllium powder, baking powder, and salt.
4. Mix until well incorporated, let the batter rest three to four minutes.
5. Prep/plug in your waffle maker to preheat.
6. Spread half of the batter on the waffle maker and cook for three to four minutes. Remove and set it on a cooling rack.
7. Cook the second half of batter and remove it to cool.
8. Once cool, assemble the chaffles with the marshmallow fluff and chocolate, using two tablespoons of marshmallow and ¼ bar of Lily's Chocolate.
9. Eat as is, or toast for a melty - gooey S'more sandwich.

Vanilla Twinkie Chaffle

Servings Provided: 6

Nutritional Facts - Per Serving:

- Net Carbohydrates: 6.5 grams
- Calories: 152
- Protein: 6.1 grams
- Fats: 9 grams

Ingredients Needed:

- Butter - melted & cooled (2 tbsp.)
- Unchilled cream cheese - softened (2 oz.)
- Unchilled eggs (2 large)
- Vanilla extract (1 tsp.)
- Optional: Vanilla Cupcake Extract (.5 tsp.)
- Lakanto Confectioners (.25 cup)
- Pinch of pink salt
- Almond flour (.25 cup)
- Coconut flour (2 tbsp.)
- Baking powder (1 tsp.)

Preparation Directions:

1. Preheat a Corn Dog Maker.

2. Melt the butter and let it cool a minute. Whisk the eggs into the butter until creamy. Add vanilla, extract, sweetener, salt, and then blend well.
3. Fold in the almond flour, coconut flour, and baking powder. Blend until well incorporated.
4. Add two tablespoons of the batter to each well and spread across evenly.
5. Close the lid to cook for four minutes.
6. Remove and cool on a rack.

Walnut Low-Carb Chaffles

Servings Provided: 2

Nutritional Facts - Per Serving:

- Net Carbohydrates: 1.03 grams
- Calories: 95
- Protein: 2.94 grams
- Fats: 8.93 grams

Ingredients Needed:

- Cream cheese (2 tbsp.)
- Almond flour (.5 tsp.)
- Baking powder (.25 tsp.)
- Chopped walnuts (.25 cup)
- Stevia extract powder (1 pinch)
- Egg (1 large)

Preparation Directions:

1. Warm the mini waffle iron and spray it with a misting of cooking oil spray.
2. Whisk the fixings and spoon the batter into the maker to cook for two to three minutes.
3. Let them cool for a few minutes before serving.

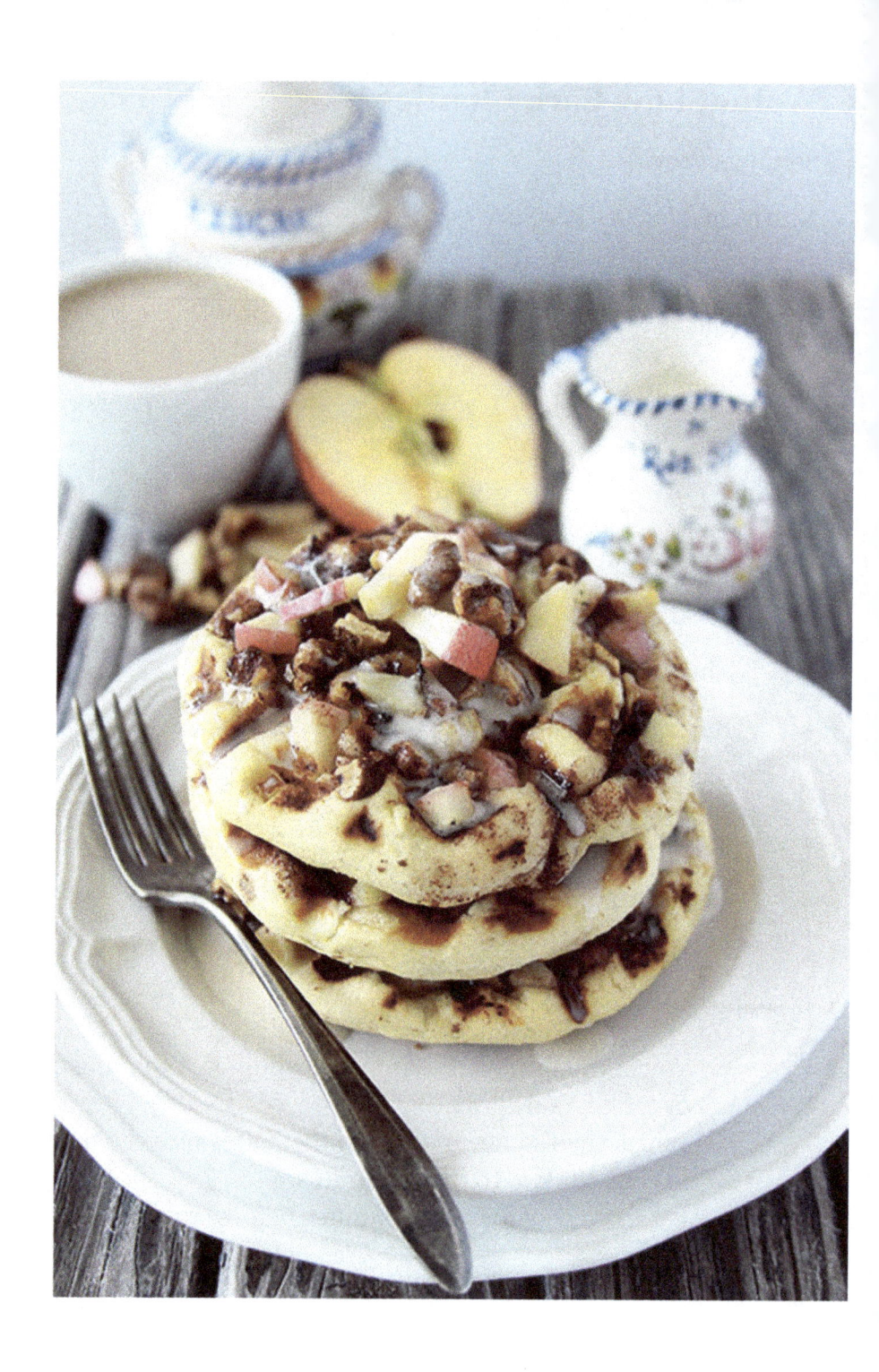

Caramel Cake

Yields Provided: 12 Servings

Macro Counts for Each Serving:

- Total Net Carbs: 4.2 g
- Fat Content: 34.9 g
- Protein: 9.5 g
- Calories: 388

List of Ingredients:

- Almond flour (2.5 cups)
- Coconut flour (.25 cup)
- Unflavored whey protein powder (.25 cup)
- Salt (.5 tsp.)
- Baking powder (1 tbsp.)
- Softened butter (.5 cup)
- Swerve sweetener (.66 cup)
- Eggs - room temperature (4 large)
- Vanilla extract (1 tsp.)
- Almond milk (.75 cup)
- Sugar-free caramel sauce (2 batches)

Preparation Technique - The Cake:

1. Set the oven to 325° Fahrenheit. Grease two 8-inch round cake pans. Cut a sheet of parchment to line the bottoms of the pans and grease the parchment as well.

2. Sift the coconut and almond flour, whey protein, salt, and baking powder.
3. Beat the butter and sweetener until light and fluffy. Beat in the eggs - one at a time and scrape down the beaters and bowl as needed. Fold in the vanilla extract.
4. Fold in the dry fixings in two additions; alternating with the almond milk. Beat until well combined.
5. Scoop the batter into the two cake pans; spreading it evenly to the edges. Smooth the tops and bake until the tops are firm to the touch (25 min.).
6. Place on the countertop to cool while in the pans. Then, flip out onto a wire rack. Be sure to peel off the parchment paper if it sticks to the cake layers.

Preparation Technique - Caramel Glaze:

1. Prepare a double batch of the Sugar-Free Caramel Sauce but DO NOT add the additional water at the end of the recipe. Be sure to use a large saucepan (at least 3-quarts) as it will bubble up.
2. Let the sauce cool down to room temperature. It should be quite thick at this point, but still pourable, and it will continue to thicken as it cools.
3. Place one layer of cake on a serving platter and pour about one-third of the caramel sauce on top. Carefully spread to the edges with an offset spatula and let sit another 10 to 15 minutes to thicken further.
4. Secure layer two and pour some of the caramel over the top, letting it drip down the sides, spreading it over the top and sides as you go. Continue until the top and sides are well covered. Alternatively, you can

simply let it drip down the sides and not spread it over.

5. ***If your caramel is too thin and is dripping too much off the sides of the cake, you can whisk in a tablespoon or two of powdered Swerve to help thicken it up. If it gets too thick, you can gently rewarm it over low heat to thin it up again.

Carrot & Apple Spice Walnut Cake

Yields Provided: 8 Servings

Macro Counts for Each Serving:

- Fat Content: 25 g
- Total Net Carbs: 4 g
- Protein: 6 g
- Calories: 268

List of Ingredients:

- Eggs (3)
- Apple pie spice (1.5 tsp.)
- Almond flour (1 cup)
- Swerve (.66 cup)
- Baking powder (1 tsp.)
- Coconut oil (.25 cup)
- Shredded carrots (1 cup)
- Heavy whipping cream (.5 cup)
- Chopped walnuts (.5 cup)
- Also Needed: 6-inch cake pan

Preparation Technique:

1. Grease the cake pan.
2. Combine all of the fixings with the mixer until well incorporated. Pour into the pan and cover with a layer of foil.

3. Pour two cups of water into the Instant Pot bowl along with the steamer rack.
4. Arrange the pan on the trivet and set the pot using the cake button (40 min.).
5. Natural release the pressure for ten minutes, and quick release the rest of the built-up pressure.
6. Place on a rack to cool before frosting. You can also eat it plain.

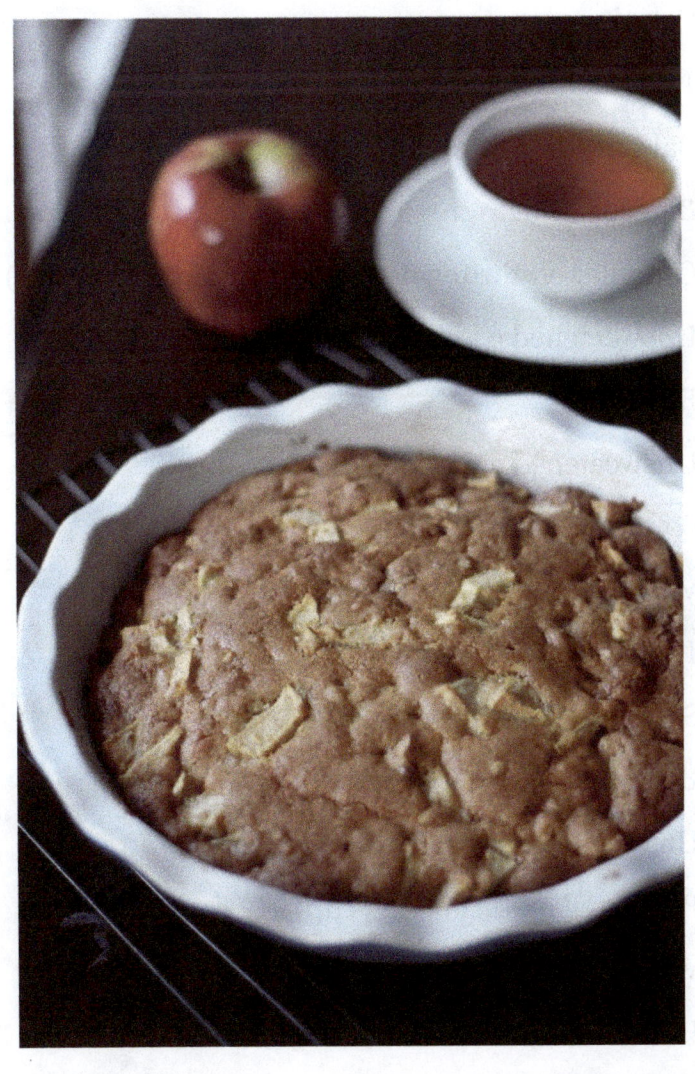

Chocolate-Lovers Cake

Yields Provided: 16 Servings

Macro Counts for Each Serving:

- Fat Content: 22.7 g
- Total Net Carbs: 5 g
- Protein: 5.9g
- Calories:252

List of Ingredients - The Cake:

- Baking powder (1 tsp.)
- Blanched finely ground almond flour (2 cups)
- Granular erythritol, or preferred sweetener (1 cup)
- Unsweetened cocoa powder (.5 cup)
- Eggs (2)
- Unsweetened almond milk (1 cup)
- Softened butter (.5 cup)
- Vanilla extract (1 tsp.)

List of Ingredients - The Frosting:

- Softened cream cheese (8 oz.)
- Butter - softened (.5 cup)
- Unsweetened cocoa powder (3 tbsp.)
- Powdered erythritol (.33 cup)
- Vanilla extract (1 tsp.)
- Heavy whipping cream (2 tbsp.)

- Optional: Lily's Chocolate Chips (for drizzling and sprinkling around edges)
- Also Needed: 6-inch round cake pans (3)

Preparation Technique:

1. Warm the oven to 350° Fahrenheit.
2. Whisk the erythritol, almond flour, cocoa powder, and baking powder until fully combined in a mixing container. Fold in the butter and vanilla.
3. Whisk the eggs into the bowl, mixing well. Pour in the almond milk.
4. Prepare the cake pans or work in batches if needed. Spritz the pans with a layer of cooking oil spray to prevent sticking. Dump the batter into the pans.
5. Bake until it springs back when you touch in the center (20-25 min.).
6. Cool completely before removing from the pan or it may fall apart. For best results, cool to room temperature for a few hours.
7. Prepare the Frosting: Whip all ingredients together until fluffy, 3-5 minutes.
1. 8. To assemble: Place the first layer of the cake on a work surface. Spread ⅓ of the frosting over top. Arrange the middle cake layer and add frosting, repeat and smooth frosting over top.
8. Add any optional toppings or drizzles to your liking.

Instant Pot Orange Rum Cake

Yields Provided: 6 Servings

Macro Counts for Each Serving:

- Fat Content: 22 g
- Total Net Carbs: 4 g
- Protein: 7 g
- Calories: 262

List of Ingredients:

- Eggs (3)
- Baking powder (2 tsp.)
- Almond flour (1.5 cups)
- Butter - softened (.5 cup)
- Coconut flour (.5 cup)
- Orange extract (1 tsp.)
- Xanthan gum (.25 tsp.)
- Salt (1 pinch)
- Granulated erythritol sweetener (.75 cup or as desired)
- Almond milk (1 cup)
- Gold rum (3 tbsp.)
- Orange zest (1 tsp.)

Preparation Technique:

1. Combine in a blender; the eggs, zest, orange extract, gold rum, almond milk, erythritol, and the butter.

2. Blend for 1 minute and add the rest of the fixings (Baking powder, almond flour, xanthan gum, coconut flour, and salt). Blend an additional 20 seconds.
3. Grease the pan to fit inside the Instant Pot on the trivet. Pour in 1 cup of water and secure the lid.
4. Use the high-pressure setting (8 min.).
5. Quick-release the pressure and open the lid to cool for about ten minutes before serving.

Keto Vanilla Pound Cake

Yields Provided: 12 Servings

Macro Counts for Each Serving:

- Total Net Carbs: 5.23 g
- Fat Content: 20.67 g
- Protein: 7.67 g
- Calories: 249

List of Ingredients:

- Almond flour (2 cups)
- Baking powder (2 tsp.)
- Granular erythritol - Swerve (1 cup)
- Sour cream (1 cup)
- Butter (.5 cup)
- Cream cheese (2 oz.)
- Large eggs (4)
- Vanilla extract (1 tsp.)
- Also Needed: 9-inch Bundt pan

Preparation Technique:

1. Set the oven to 350° Fahrenheit
2. Generously butter the pan and set aside
3. Sift the baking powder and almond flour in a bowl, and place it to the side for now.
4. Dice the butter into several squares and toss into a separate bowl with the cream cheese. Microwave for 30 seconds. Stir until well combined.

5. Add the sour cream, erythritol, vanilla extract to the mixture. Stir well.
6. Pour the wet fixings into the large bowl of flour and baking powder. Stir well, adding the eggs to the batter. Stir well and empty into the baking pan.
7. Bake for 50 minutes.
8. For best results, let the cake cool completely for at least two hours, preferably overnight. If you remove it too soon, it may crumble a somewhat.

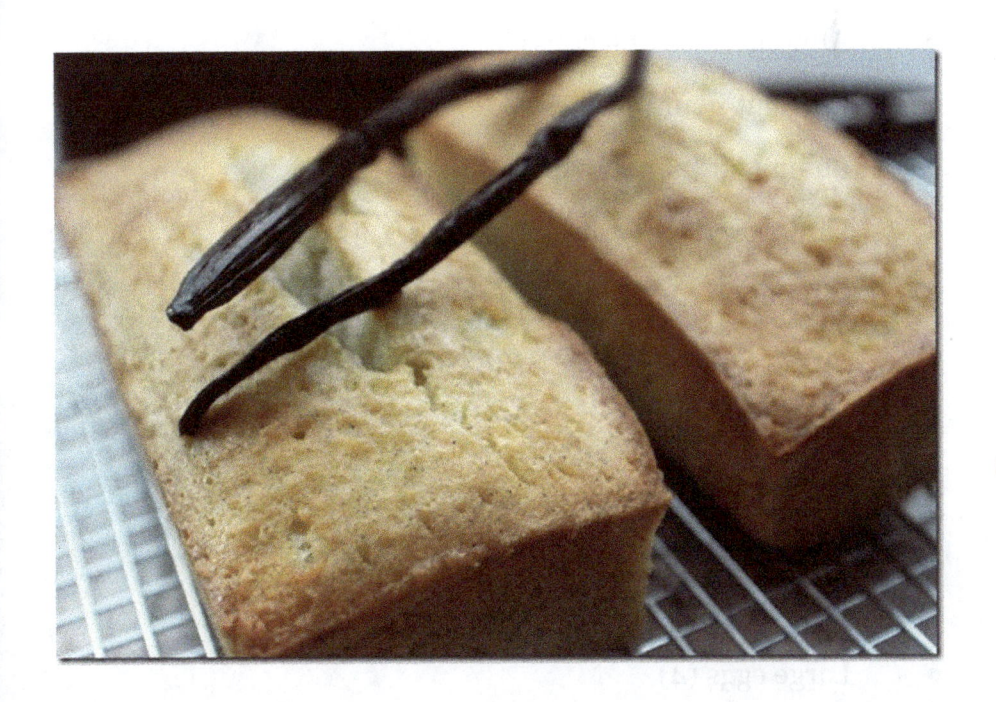

Pumpkin Caramel Bundt Cake

Yields Provided: 16 Servings

Macro Counts for Each Serving:

- Total Net Carbs: 5 g
- Fat Content: 16.5 g
- Protein: 8 g
- Calories: 212

List of Ingredients - For the Cake:

- Almond flour (2.5 cups)
- Coconut flour (.5 cup)
- Baking powder (1 tbsp.)
- Unflavored whey protein powder (.33 cup)
- Cinnamon (2 tsp.)
- Swerve sweetener (.66 cup)
- Ginger (1 tsp.)
- Salt (.5 tsp.)
- Cloves (.25 tsp.)
- Pumpkin puree (1.5 cups)
- Large eggs (4)
- Melted butter (.25 cup)
- Water (.5 to .66 cup)
- Vanilla extract (1 tsp.)

List of Ingredients - For the Glaze:

- Pure molasses (1 tsp.)
- Butter (.25 cup)
- Powdered Swerve sweetener (.5 cup)
- Caramel flavor (.5 tsp.)
- Whipping cream (2 tbsp.)
- 9-inch Bundt pan

Preparation - Technique - Cake Preparation:

1. Warm up the oven to 325° Fahrenheit.
2. Grease the pan well.
3. Whisk the baking powder, almond flour, Swerve, salt, protein powder, cloves, and ginger in the mixing bowl.
4. Fold in the eggs, pumpkin puree, .5 cup water, butter, and vanilla extract. Add small amounts of water as needed for a thick consistency.
5. Empty the batter into the greased pan.
6. Bake 55 to 60 minutes. Test for doneness.
7. Remove and let cool 15 minutes.
8. Place onto the rack to cool.

Preparation - Technique - The Glaze:

1. Use the low heat setting in a saucepan to melt the butter and molasses. Stir well.
2. Take the pan off the burner and add in the caramel extract, powdered sweetener, and whipping cream.
3. Drizzle over the cake and serve.

Pumpkin Pie Spice Mug Cake

Yields Provided: 4 Servings

Macro Counts for Each Serving:

- Fat Content: 12 g
- Total Net Carbs: 4 g
- Protein: 8 g
- Calories: 166

List of Ingredients:

- Heavy whipping cream (.25 cup)
- Pumpkin puree (.5 cup)
- Classic monk fruit sweetener (4 tbsp. - divided)
- Eggs (4)
- Pure vanilla extract (.5 tsp.)
- Baking soda (.5 tsp.)
- Coconut flour (.25 cup + 1 tbsp.)
- Cream of tartar (1 tsp.)
- Ground allspice (.25 tsp.)
- Cinnamon (.75 tsp. - divided)
- Ground cloves (.125 tsp.)
- Ginger (.25 tsp.)
- Nutmeg (.25 tsp.)
- Nonstick cooking spray

Preparation Technique:

1. Add 2 tbsp. monk fruit sweetener and heavy cream into a mixing container. Whip using the high setting with an electric mixer. Cover with a lid or plastic wrap and chill in the fridge.

2. Add the eggs, pumpkin puree, and vanilla extract into a mixing container. Blend using an electric mixer until well mixed and smooth.
3. Add the remaining 2 tbsp. sweetener, baking soda, cream of tartar, coconut flour, ginger, nutmeg, .5 tsp. cinnamon, allspice, and cloves. Mix well.
4. Coat the four coffee mugs with a spritz of nonstick cooking spray. Spoon ¼ of the pumpkin batter into each mug. Microwave one-by-one until the cakes are done (2 min.).
5. Serve with a dollop of whipped cream, and a sprinkle of cinnamon.

Slow-Cooked Gingerbread Cake

Yields Provided: 10 Servings

Macro Counts for Each Serving:

- Fat Content: 25 g
- Total Net Carbs: 8.6 g
- Protein: 9 g
- Calories: 223

List of Ingredients:

- Almond or sunflower seed flour (2.25 cups)
- Coconut flour (2 tbsp.)
- Swerve sweetener (.75 cup)
- Ground ginger (1.5 tbsp.)
- Dark cocoa powder (1 tbsp.)
- Ground cinnamon (.5 tbsp.)
- Salt (.25 tsp.)
- Baking powder (2 tsp.)
- Ground cloves (.5 tsp.)
- Melted butter (.5 cup)
- Vanilla extract (1 tsp.)
- Water or almond milk (.66 cup)
- Lemon juice (1 tbsp.)
- Suggested Size Cooker: 6-quarts

Preparation Technique:

1. Prepare the cooker with a portion of cooking spray or oil.
2. Whisk all of the flour, salt, cloves, baking powder, ginger, cinnamon, sweetener, and cocoa powder.
3. Blend in the almond milk/water, melted butter, eggs, vanilla extract, and lemon juice.
4. Empty the batter into the slow cooker and cook until set – approximately 2.5 to 3 hours.
5. Garnish as desired and enjoy, but count those carbs.

Tiramisu Layer Cake

Yields Provided: 10 Servings

Macro Counts for Each Serving:

- Fat Content: 38 g
- Total Net Carbs: 5 g
- Protein: 9 g
- Calories: 408

List of Ingredients - The Cake:

- Baking powder (1 tsp.)
- Blanched almond flour (1.5 cups)
- Erythritol (.5 cup)
- Sea salt (.125 tsp.)
- Unchilled softened butter (.33 cup)
- Unchilled eggs (3 large)
- Unchilled heavy cream (.25 cup)
- Vanilla extract (1 tsp.)
- Also Needed: 9-inch baking pan

List of Ingredients - The Drizzle:

- Espresso/strong coffee - at room temperature (.25 cup)
- Brandy or cognac (2 tbsp. optional)

List of Ingredients - The Filling:

- Unchilled egg yolks (4 large)
- Powdered erythritol (.25 cup)

- Unchilled Mascarpone (1 cup)
- Cold heavy cream (1 cup)
- Cocoa powder (optional for dusting (.5 tsp.)

Preparation Technique - The Cake:

1. Set the oven temperature to 350° Fahrenheit. Prepare the pan with parchment baking paper, so that it hangs over the sides.
2. Mix/whisk together the erythritol and butter until combined.
3. Whisk and add the eggs, vanilla extract, and heavy cream.
4. Beat in the salt, almond flour, and baking powder until smooth.
5. Transfer the dough to the lined pan. Bake for 20 to 25 minutes until firm.

Preparation Technique - The Filling:

1. Prepare a double boiler with boiling water. Combine the egg yolks and powdered sweetener into the top of the pan. Reduce the heat setting to low, and simmer for about 7 to 10 minutes, stirring constantly, until it has increased in volume and is a little frothy.
2. Remove from the heat. Use a hand mixer using the med-low speed to whip the yolks until they're thick and lemon in color. Set aside to cool.
3. In another container, whip the heavy cream using the high-speed until stiff peaks are formed.
4. Add the mascarpone to the prepared yolks, beating at the low-speed until combined.
5. Fold the mascarpone yolk mixture in with the whipped cream.
1. Preparation Technique - The Assembly:

1. Use a butter knife if needed to remove the cake from the edges of the pan. Transfer to a cutting board.
2. Whisk the espresso and brandy. Drizzle evenly over the cake.
3. Cut the cake in half, forming two rectangles. Carefully slide one half onto a platter.
4. Top the cake on the platter with half of the cream mixture. Carefully place the second half of the cake on top, then top with the remaining cream mixture.
5. Sift cocoa powder through a fine-mesh sieve over the tiramisu (optional).
6. Refrigerate for 4 hours, or preferably overnight, to set.

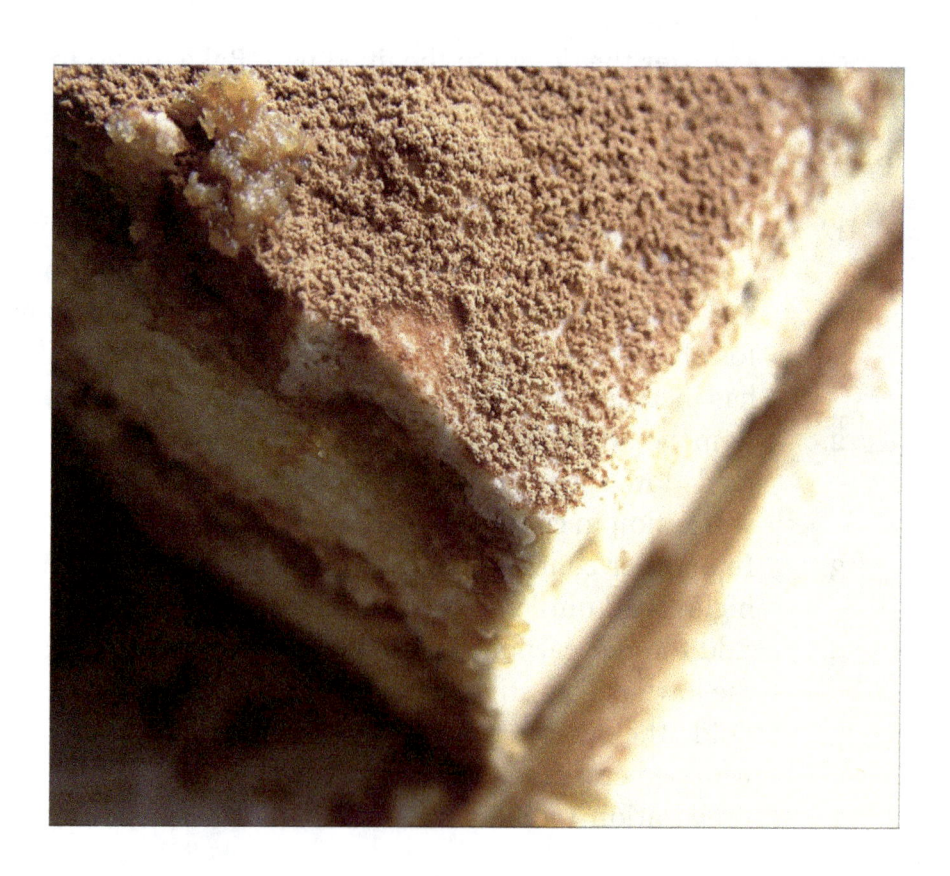

No-Bake Banana Split Cheesecake

Yields Provided: 20 Servings Macro Counts for Each Serving:

- Fat Content: 30 g
- Total Net Carbs: 6.7 g
- Protein: 4.1 g
- Calories: 302

List of Ingredients - The Crust:

- Cinnamon (2 tsp.)
- Almond flour (3 cups)
- Swerve (.33 cup)
- Melted butter (1 cup)
- Also Needed: 9 x 13-inch pan

List of Ingredients - The Filling:

- Swerve confectioner's sugar (1 cup)
- Melted butter (1 cup)
- Cream cheese (16 oz.)

List of Ingredients – The Topping:

- Chopped banana (1)
- Sliced strawberries (2 pints)
- Lemon juice (1 tbsp.)
- Heavy whipping cream (2 cups)
- Gelatin (1.5 tsp.)
- Vanilla extract (1 tsp.)

- Swerve (3 tbsp.)
- Water (3 tbsp.)
- Optional: Chocolate sauce & Nuts

Preparation Technique:

1. Combine the crust fixings and press together in the pan.
2. Melt the butter and mix with the sweetener and cream cheese until creamy. Spread on top of the crust.
3. Combine the strawberries and banana in a mixing dish along with the lemon juice. Make the next layer.
4. Prepare the topping. Combine the whipping cream and gelatin in the water and beat well. Blend in the vanilla extract and sweetener. Whip until it is creamy to cover and make the next layer.
5. Top with the chocolate sauce and nuts if you like it that way.

No-Bake Plain Cheesecake

Yields Provided: 6 Servings

Macro Counts for Each Serving:

- Fat Content: 25 g
- Total Net Carbs: 5 g
- Protein: 6.9 g
- Calories: 247

List of Ingredients - The Crust:

- Melted coconut oil (2 tbsp.)
- Almond flour (2 tbsp.)
- Swerve Confectioner's/equivalent (2 tbsp.)
- Crushed salted almonds (2 tbsp.)

List of Ingredients - The Filling:

- Swerve confectioner's/equivalent (.25 cup)
- Gelatin (1 tsp.)
- Cream cheese (16 oz. pkg.)
- Unsweetened almond milk (.5 cup)
- Vanilla extract (1 tsp.)

Preparation Technique:

1. Prepare the crust by combining all of the fixings under the crust section. Place one heaping tablespoon into the bottom of dessert cups. Press the mixture down and set aside.

2. Prepare the filling. Mix the sweetener and gelatin. Pour in the milk and stir (5 min.). Whip the vanilla beans and cream cheese with a mixer on medium until creamy. Add the gelatin mixture slowly until well incorporated.
3. Pour the mixture over the crust of each cup. Chill for three hours, minimum.

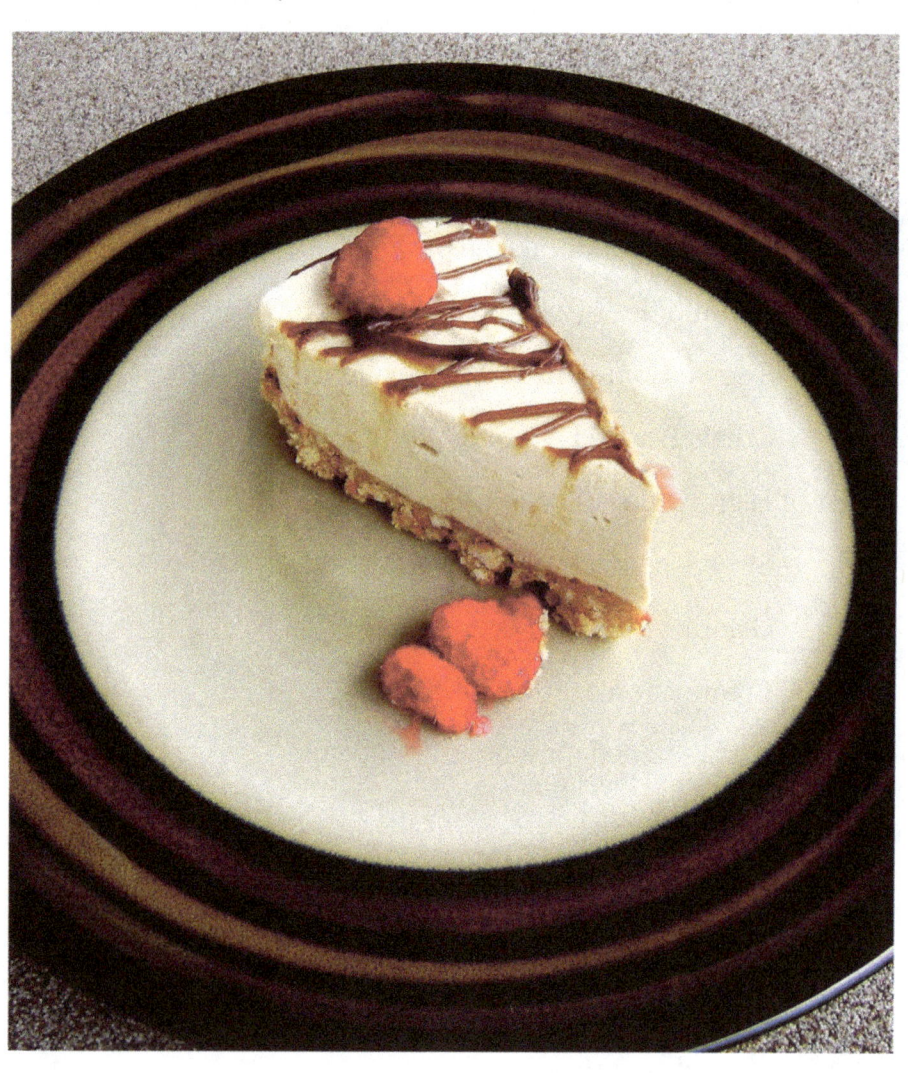

Almond Cinnamon Butter Cookies

Yields Provided: 12 Servings

Macro Counts for Each Serving:

- Total Net Carbs: 10.4 g
- Fat Content: 18.4 g
- Protein: 5 g
- Calories: 196

List of Ingredients:

- Blanched almond flour (2 cups)
- Softened butter (.5 cup)
- Egg (1)
- Ground cinnamon (1 tsp.)
- Low-calorie natural sweetener - Swerve (.5 cup)
- Sugar-free vanilla extract (1 tsp.)

Preparation Technique:

1. Set the oven temperature to 350° Fahrenheit. Cover a cookie sheet with a layer of parchment baking paper.
2. Combine the almond flour, butter, egg, sweetener, vanilla extract, and cinnamon in mixing container. Stir well to prepare the dough.
3. Separate the dough into one-inch balls. Arrange in the baking sheet and press with a fork in a crisscross pattern.
4. Bake until edges are golden (12 to 15 minutes). Cool on the baking tray for one minute before removing to a cooling rack.

Amaretti Cookies

Yields Provided: 16 Servings

Macro Counts for Each Serving:

- Total Net Carbs: 1 g
- Protein: 2.5 g
- Fat Content: 8 g
- Calories: 86

List of Ingredients:

- Coconut flour (2 tbsp.)
- Cinnamon (.25 tsp.)
- Salt (.5 tsp.)
- Erythritol (.5 cup)
- Baking powder (.5 tsp.)
- Almond flour (1 cup)
- Eggs (2)
- Almond extract (.5 tsp.)
- Vanilla extract (.5 tsp.)
- Coconut oil (4 tbsp.)
- Sugar-free jam (2 tbsp.)
- Shredded coconut (1 tbsp.)

Preparation Technique:

1. Cover the tin with a sheet of paper.
2. Warm up the oven to reach 400° Fahrenheit.

3. Sift the flour and combine all of the dry fixings.
4. After combined, work in the wet ones. Shape into 16 cookies.
5. Make a dent in the center of each one. Bake for 15 to 17 minutes.
6. It's important to let them cool for a few minutes.
7. Add a dab of jam to each one and a sprinkle of the coconut bits.

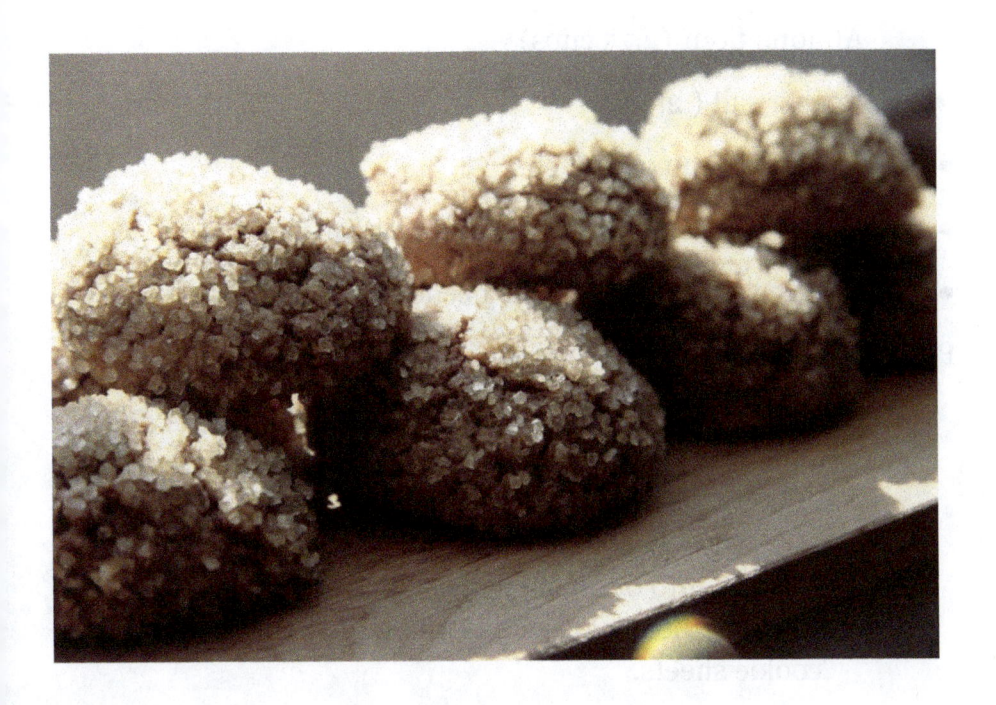

Chocolate Chip Cookies

Yields Provided: 18 Servings

Macro Counts for Each Serving:

- Fat Content: 9 g
- Total Net Carbs: 1g
- Protein: 2 g
- Calories: 96

List of Ingredients:

- Eggs (2 large)
- Grass-fed melted butter (1 stick - .5 cup)
- Heavy cream (2 tbsp.)
- Alcohol-free pure vanilla extract (2 tsp.)
- Almond flour (2.75 cups)
- Kosher salt (.25 tsp.)
- Swerve (.5 cup or to taste)
- Dark chocolate chips - ex. Lily's (.75 cup)
- Cooking spray (spritz or as needed)

Preparation Technique:

1. Warm the oven to 350° Fahrenheit. Prepare the pan.
2. Whisk the egg with the heavy cream, butter, vanilla, almond flour, salt, and swerve.
3. Fold the chocolate chips into the batter. Form the mixture into one-inch balls.
4. Arrange the cookies about three inches apart onto the cookie sheets.

5. Bake about 17 to 19 minutes. Cool slightly to enjoy.

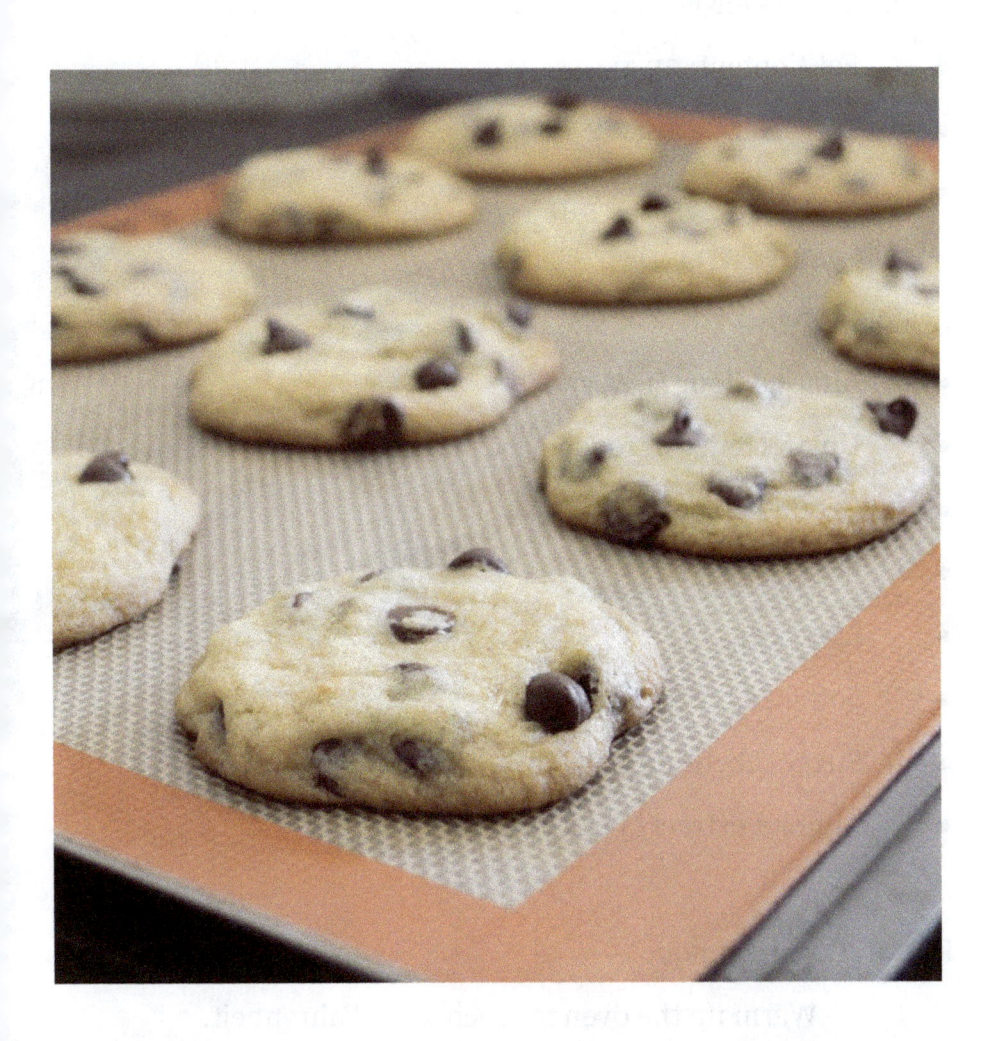

Coconut Cookies

Yields Provided: 6 Servings

Macro Counts for Each Serving:
- Fat Content: 25 g
- Total Net Carbs: 2 g
- Protein: 7 g
- Calories: 271

List of Ingredients:
- Almond flour (1.25 cups)
- Unsweetened shredded coconut (.5 cup)
- Ground cinnamon (.25 tsp.)
- Sea salt (.25 tsp.)
- Large eggs (3)
- Softened butter (6 tbsp.)
- Sugar substitute (.33 cup)
- Almond extract (1 tsp.)

Preparation Technique:
1. Warm up the oven to reach 350° Fahrenheit.
2. Spritz a baking tin with some cooking oil spray.
3. Combine the sweetener of choice and softened butter.
4. One at a time; whisk and stir in the three eggs until well mixed.

5. Stir in the rest of the fixings – with the coconut added last.
6. Drop the cookie mixture by spoonful onto the cookie sheet. Bake for 10 to 15 minutes. Cool before storing.

Cranberry Bliss Cookies

Yields Provided: 18 Servings

Macro Counts for Each Serving:

- Total Net Carbs: 2.05 g
- Fat Content: 13.15 g
- Protein: 3.3 g
- Calories: 145

List of Ingredients - The Cookies:

- Almond flour (2 cups)
- Swerve Sweetener (.5 cup)
- Baking powder (1 tsp.)
- Ground ginger (.75 tsp.)
- Salt (.25 tsp.)
- Softened butter (6 tbsp.)
- Unchilled egg room (1 large)
- Vanilla extract (.5 tsp.)
- Fresh cranberries (.25 cup - chopped)

List of Ingredients - The Frosting:

- Cream cheese - softened (4 oz.)
- Powdered Swerve Sweetener (2 tbsp.)
- Melted cocoa butter or melted coconut oil (.5 oz.)
- Vanilla extract (.25 tsp.)

- Unsweetened finely chopped fresh cranberries (.25 cup) or freeze-dried cranberries crushed

List of Ingredients - The Drizzle:

- Cocoa butter melted/coconut oil (.5 oz.)
- Powdered Swerve Sweetener (2 tbsp.)

Preparation Technique:

1. Warm the oven to in advance to reach 325° Fahrenheit.
2. Prepare a large baking tray with a layer of parchment baking paper.
3. Whisk the baking powder, almond flour, salt, and ginger. In a large mixing container, mix the sweetener and butter until well combined. Fold in the vanilla extract and whisked egg.
4. Mix in the dry fixings and fold in the chopped cranberries.
5. Scoop and roll into one-inch balls. Press flat (.33-inch thickness) on the tin a few inches apart.
6. Bake 12 to 15 minutes until not quite firm to the touch. They will firm up as they sit. Let cool on pan.
7. Prepare the Frosting: Beat the cream cheese with powdered sweetener until well combined. Melt and slowly add the cocoa butter and vanilla extract.
8. Frost the cookies. Decorate with a sprinkle of dried cranberries.
9. Whisk the powdered sweetener and melted cocoa butter until smooth. Drizzle over the cookies and let them sit for half an hour before serving.

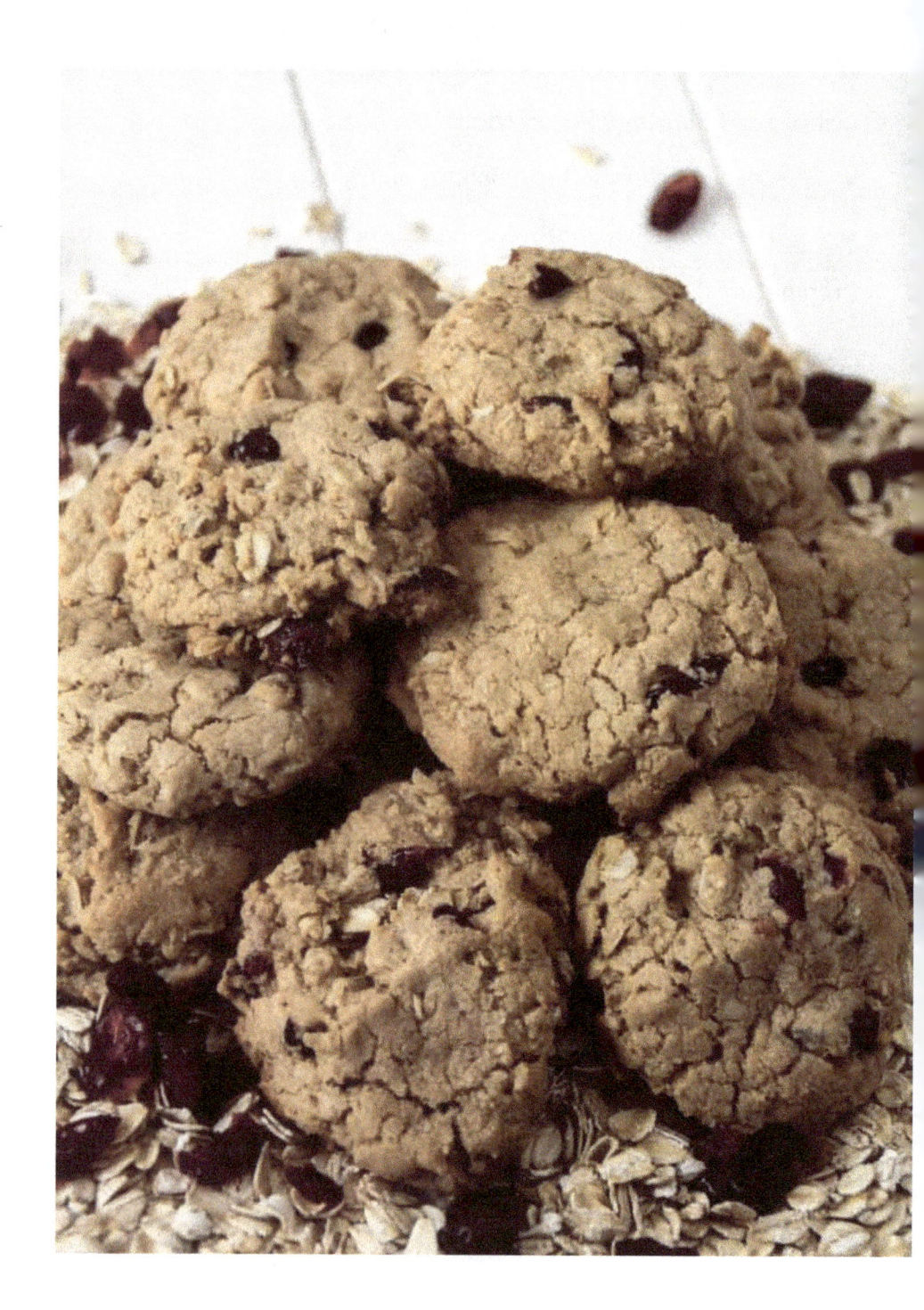

CPSIA information can be obtained
at www.ICGtesting.com
Printed in the USA
BVHW061924220321
603177BV00010B/813

9 781801 901758